Manual of Undergraduate Psychiatric Education

Manual of Undergraduate Psychiatric Education

Edited by

Marsal Sanches, M.D., Ph.D.

Michael McClam, M.D.

Robert Boland, M.D.

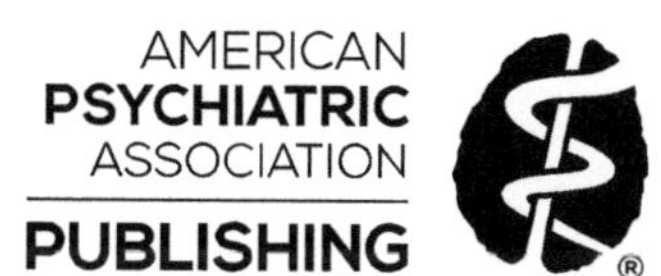

Note: The authors have worked to ensure that all information in this book is accurate at the time of publication and consistent with general psychiatric and medical standards, and that information concerning drug dosages, schedules, and routes of administration is accurate at the time of publication and consistent with standards set by the U.S. Food and Drug Administration and the general medical community. As medical research and practice continue to advance, however, therapeutic standards may change. Moreover, specific situations may require a specific therapeutic response not included in this book. For these reasons and because human and mechanical errors sometimes occur, we recommend that readers follow the advice of physicians directly involved in their care or the care of a member of their family.

Books published by American Psychiatric Association Publishing represent the findings, conclusions, and views of the individual authors and do not necessarily represent the policies and opinions of American Psychiatric Association Publishing or the American Psychiatric Association.

First Edition

Manufactured in the United States of America on acid-free paper
29 28 27 26 25 5 4 3 2 1
American Psychiatric Association Publishing
800 Maine Avenue SW, Suite 900 Washington, DC 20024–2812 www.appi.org

Library of Congress Cataloging-in-Publication Data
Names: Sanches, Marsal editor | McClam, Michael editor | Boland, Robert Joseph editor Title: Manual of undergraduate psychiatric education / edited by Marsal Sanches, Michael McClam, Robert Boland.Description: First edition. | Washington, DC : American Psychiatric Association Publishing, [2025] | Includes bibliographical references and index. Identifiers: LCCN 2025024618 (print) | LCCN 2025024619 (ebook) | ISBN 9798894551142 paperback | ISBN 9798894551159 ebook Subjects: LCSH: Psychiatry--Study and teaching--United States Classification: LCC RC336 .M33 2025 (print) | LCC RC336 (ebook) LC record available at https://lccn.loc.gov/2025024618 LC ebook record available at https://lccn.loc.gov/2025024619

British Library Cataloguing in Publication Data
A CIP record is available from the British Library.

EU GPSR Authorized Representative: LOGOS EUROPE, 9 rue Nicolas Poussin, 17000, LA ROCHELLE, France; E-mail: Contact@logoseurope.eu

Contents

Part II: Practical Aspects of Undergraduate Psychiatric Education

Part III: Teaching Techniques

Contributors

Andrew R. Alkis, M.D.
Clinical Assistant Professor, College of Medicine and Department of Psychiatry and Behavioral Sciences, Medical University of South Carolina, Mount Pleasant, South Carolina

Hermioni L. Amonoo, M.D., M.P.P., M.P.H.
Associate Professor, Department of Psychiatry, Harvard Medical School; Associate Program Director, Brigham and Women's Hospital; Attending Physician, Dana-Farber Cancer Institute, Boston, Massachusetts

Khalid Bazaid, M.D.
Chair, Canadian Academy of CAP Education Committee; Assistant Professor, Department of Psychiatry, University of Ottawa; Child and Adolescent Psychiatrist, Youth Psychiatry Program, Royal Ottawa Mental Health Centre, University of Ottawa, Ottawa, Ontario, Canada

Abdellah Bezzahou, M.D.
Attending Psychiatrist, University of Manitoba, Winnipeg, Manitoba, Canada

Robert Boland, M.D.
Senior Vice President and Chief of Staff, The Menninger Clinic; Professor and Vice Chair, Menninger Department of Psychiatry and Behavioral Sciences, Baylor College of Medicine, Houston, Texas

Adam M. Brenner, M.D.
Professor of Psychiatry, Distinguished Teaching Professor, Director of Adult Psychiatry Residency Training, and Vice Chair for Education in Psychiatry, University of Texas Southwestern Medical Center, Dallas, Texas

Amy S. Brenner, M.S.W., LCSW-S
Adjunct Assistant Professor, UTSouthwestern Medical Center School of Health Professions; Clinical Therapist, Dallas Texas

Carlyle H. Chan, M.D.
Professor and Vice Chair, Professional Development and Educational Outreach, Department of Psychiatry and Behavioral Medicine, Medical College of Wisconsin, Milwaukee, Wisconsin

Helen L. Dainton-Howard, M.D.
Fellow, Rush University, Chicago, Illinois

Shaheen A. Darani, M.D.
Assistant Professor, Department of Psychiatry, University of Toronto, Toronto, Ontario, Canada

Steven A. Epstein, M.D.
Professor and Physician Executive Director, MedStar Behavioral Health Professor and Chair, Department of Psychiatry, Georgetown University School of Medicine, Washington, DC

J. Chase Findley, M.D.
Associate Professor, McGovern Medical School at UTHealth Houston, Houston, Texas

Jin Y. Han, M.D.
Associate Professor, Psychiatry Clerkship Director and Sub-Internship Director, Menninger Department of Psychiatry and Behavioral Sciences, Baylor College of Medicine, Houston, Texas

Pochu Ho, M.D.
Assistant Professor of Psychiatry, Yale University; Director of Psychiatric Consultation Service, West Haven VA Medical Center, New Haven, Connecticut

Poh Choo How, M.D., Ph.D.
Associate Clinical Professor, University of California, Davis, Sacramento, California

Sindhu A. Idicula, M.D.
Associate Professor, Associate Training Director, and Director of Psychotherapy Education, Department of Psychiatry and Behavioral Sciences, Baylor College of Medicine, Houston, Texas

Laura Kenyon, M.D.
Psychiatry Resident, Department of Psychiatry and Behavioral Sciences, Baylor College of Medicine, Houston, Texas

Elijah Li, M.D.
Medical Student, Baylor College of Medicine, Houston, Texas

John Luo, M.D.
Health Sciences Clinical Professor of Psychiatry and Human Behavior, University of California, Irvine School of Medicine, Orange, California

Anuron Mandal, M.D.
Assistant Professor, Department of Psychiatry and Behavioral Sciences, Baylor College of Medicine; Attending Psychiatrist, The Menninger Clinic, Houston, Texas

Michael McClam, M.D.
Assistant Professor, Menninger Department of Psychiatry, Baylor College of Medicine, Houston, Texas

Enoch Ng, M.D., Ph.D.
Attending Psychiatrist, Sunnybrook Health Sciences Centre, Toronto, Ontario, Canada

Jamie S. Padmore, D.M.
Professor and Vice Dean for Education, Georgetown University Medical Center; Vice President Academic Affairs, MedStar Health, Washington, DC

Michelle Patriquin, Ph.D.
Associate Professor, Department of Psychiatry and Behavioral Sciences, McGovern Medical School; Co-Director of Research, John S. Dunn Behavioral Sciences Center; Assistant Dean, Digital Health and Innovation, School of Behavioral Health Sciences, UTHealth Houston, Houston, Texas

Christine M. Pelic, M.D.
Assistant Professor, Ralph H. Johnson VA Medical Center; College of Medicine, Medical University of South Carolina; and Department of Psychiatry and Behavioral Sciences, Medical University of South Carolina, Charleston, South Carolina

Christopher G. Pelic, M.D.
Professor; Associate Dean for GME Outreach; Medical Director for Telepsychiatry, College of Medicine and Department of Psychiatry and Behavioral Sciences, Medical University of South Carolina, Charleston, South Carolina

Lindsey S. Pershern, M.D.
Associate Professor, Director of Psychiatry Residency Training, Menninger Department of Psychiatry, Baylor College of Medicine, Houston, Texas

Neil V. Puri, M.D.
Assistant Professor, Department of Psychiatry and Behavioral Sciences, Baylor College of Medicine; Attending Psychiatrist, The Menninger Clinic, Houston, Texas

Jeffrey J. Rakofsky, M.D.
Assistant Professor, Department of Psychiatry and Behavioral Sciences, Emory University, Atlanta, Georgia

Kalyn Reddy, M.D., M.P.H.
Chief Resident, Department of Psychiatry and Human Behavior, University of California, Irvine School of Medicine, Orange, California

Allen C. Richert Jr., M.D.
Associate Professor of Psychiatry and Human Behavior; Director of Division of Sleep Medicine; and Director of Division of Electroconvulsive Therapy, University of Mississippi Medical Center, Jackson, Mississippi

Marsal Sanches, M.D., Ph.D.
Professor, Department of Psychiatry and Behavioral Sciences, McGovern Medical School; Attending Psychiatrist and Associate Director for Research, Dunn Behavioral Sciences Center at UTHealth Houston, Houston, Texas

Ruth S. Shim, M.D., M.P.H.
Luke and Grace Kim Professor in Cultural Psychiatry; Associate Dean for Diverse and Inclusive Education; and Professor of Clinical Psychiatry, University of California, Davis, Sacramento, California

Stuart Slavin, M.D., M.Ed.
Vice President for Well-Being, Accreditation Council for Graduate Medical Education, Chicago, Illinois

Gabriella M. Thiessen, M.D.
Fourth-Year Medical Student, McGovern Medical School at UTHealth Houston, Houston, Texas

Joshua A. Trull, D.O.
Assistant Professor of Psychiatry and Human Behavior; Director of Medical Student Clerkship, University of Mississippi Medical Center, Jackson, Mississippi

Vivian Wang, M.D.
Psychiatry Resident, Department of Psychiatry and Behavioral Sciences, Baylor College of Medicine, Houston, Texas

Serena M. Weber, M.D.
Assistant Professor, Department of Psychiatry and Behavioral Sciences, Baylor College of Medicine; Attending Psychiatrist, The Menninger Clinic, Houston, Texas

Julie Williams, M.S., M.D.
Assistant Professor, Menninger Department of Psychiatry and Behavioral Sciences, Baylor College of Medicine, Houston, Texas

Marika I. Wrzosek, M.D.
Associate Professor; Associate Vice Chair for Medical Student Education, Department of Psychiatry and Behavioral Medicine, Medical College of Wisconsin, Milwaukee, Wisconsin

Disclosures

The following contributor has indicated a financial interest in or other affiliation with a commercial supporter, manufacturer of a commercial product, and/or provider of a commercial service as listed below:

Adam Brenner

- Publication/writing honoraria: EIC, *Academic Psychiatry*
- Royalties: *Psychotherapy: A Practical Introduction*

The following contributors stated that they had no competing interests during the year preceding manuscript submission:

Andrew R. Alkis, M.D., Hermioni L. Amonoo, M.D., M.P.P., M.P.H., Khalid Bazaid, M.D., Abdellah Bezzahou, M.D., Robert Boland, M.D., Adam M. Brenner, M.D., Amy S. Brenner, M.S.W., LCSW-S, Carlyle H. Chan, M.D., Helen L. Dainton-Howard, M.D., Steven A. Epstein, M.D., J. Chase Findley, M.D., Jin Y. Han, M.D., Pochu Ho, M.D., Poh Choo How, M.D., Ph.D., Laura Kenyon, M.D., Elijah Li, M.D., John Luo, M.D., Michael McClam, M.D., Enoch Ng, M.D., Ph.D., Michelle Patriquin, Ph.D., Christine M. Pelic, M.D., Christopher G. Pelic, M.D., Lindsey S. Pershern, M.D., Neil V. Puri, M.D., Jeffrey J. Rakofsky, M.D., Kalyn Reddy, M.D., M.P.H., Marsal Sanches, M.D., Ph.D., Ruth S. Shim, M.D., M.P.H., Stuart Slavin, M.D., M.Ed., Gabriella M. Thiessen, M.D., Serena M. Weber, M.D., Julie Williams, M.S., M.D.

The following contributors did not supply information regarding disclosures:

Shaheen A. Darani, M.D., Sindhu A. Idicula, M.D., Anuron Mandal, M.D., Jamie S. Padmore, D.M., Allen C. Richert Jr., M.D., Joshua A. Trull, D.O., Vivian Wang, M.D., Marika I. Wrzosek, M.D.

Introduction

Marsal Sanches, M.D., Ph.D.
Michael McClam, M.D.
Robert Boland, M.D.

This book aims to help instruct medical student educators in the best practices for being effective teachers. The medical students we teach today are the future of medicine, and the role of a teaching physician encompasses far more than just making sure students acquire enough medical knowledge to pass licensure exams, acquire clinical skills, and become proficient physicians. As we inspire medical students to think critically, establish priorities, and serve as role models, our attitudes may have profound implications for how medicine will be practiced and perceived by society in 10, 20, or 30 years.

The last several decades have witnessed profound transformations in the practice of medicine. On the one hand, countless discoveries and technological advances have enhanced medical science. On the other hand, there is concern that excessive emphasis on the technical aspects of medical practice has relegated its human components to second place. Medicine has traditionally been defined as a mixture of science and art, and balancing those two components is a prominent challenge for medical educators.

Perhaps in no other area of medicine has this debate been as meaningful as in psychiatry. Progress in our understanding of the pathophysiology of mental disorders has blurred the limits between psychiatry, neurology, and neuroscience. Psychiatry is significantly more somatic today than it was 30 years ago, in the 1990s (the "Decade of the Brain"), and the advent of novel biological therapeutic strategies, such as numerous brain stimulation options, has made psychiatry more attractive for hard-science-inclined students. Not coincidently, interest in psychiatry among senior medical students is on the rise. That increased interest, unfortunately, has not yet been enough to ameliorate growing concerns regarding the shortage of psychiatrists in the United States (Satiani et al. 2018).

These changes and concerns are reflected in different aspects of how we teach psychiatry to medical students. Psychiatry is still in the beginning stages of incorporating simulation and other technological approaches to education (Piot et al. 2020; Younes et al. 2021). The formal integration of psychiatry and medicine has become palpable in medical school curricula. Instead of complex theories and abstract conceptualizations, there is a growing focus on the practical aspects of psychiatry, in consonance with the gradual move from knowledge-based to competency-based assessment. Those changes align with the twofold mission embraced by psychiatry educators: maintaining a pipeline of future psychiatrists, and ensuring that nonpsychiatry professionals have a solid base in mental health. After all, in the United States, primary care physicians (and not psychiatrists) are often responsible for the management of patients with mental disorders (Rotenstein et al. 2023).

In addition, psychiatry educators must ensure that their students have an integrated view of their patients. It is not possible (or desirable) to dissociate the traditional aspects of clinical psychiatry from factors such as globalization, diversity and inclusion, patient agency and autonomy, the relationship between lifestyle and mental health, the customer-centered approach to medical care, and the digital revolution.

Despite the important role of national organizations in offering career advice to senior residents and faculty interested in pursuing an academic career in psychiatry, there is still a paucity of resources aimed at providing practical guidance to psychiatric educators, especially at the undergraduate level. Developing skills and expertise can be labor-intensive for educators, and they need a guide that will jump-start that process.

This book aims to fill that role. Organized and written by national leaders in the field of psychiatric education, the *Manual of Undergraduate Psychiatric Education* provides a comprehensive yet practical view of education in psychiatry. Part I covers general topics of interest for teaching psychiatrists, including a brief overview of the historical aspects of undergraduate psychiatric education, mental health and well-being in medical student education, stigma and attitudes toward psychiatry among medical students, and fostering medical student interest in psychiatry.

In Part II, the authors discuss practical aspects of teaching in the context of undergraduate psychiatric education, such as theories of learning and their implications for teaching psychiatry, the psychiatry clerkship, the teaching of psychotherapy, research education, and assessment and feedback. Part III details contemporary themes of specific interest for psychiatry educators: clinical teaching, presentation techniques, remote learning, and simulation. Finally, Part IV contains chapters on ethicolegal aspects of psychiatric education, diversity and inclusion, leadership, and career pathways in psychiatric education.

We trust that this manual, written by educators for educators, will be of value to academic psychiatrists, prospective teaching physicians, and professionals from other areas involved in psychiatric and mental health education. We hope that it will also help honor those who dedicate themselves to the essential task of teaching psychiatry at an undergraduate level.

References

Piot M-A, Dechartres A, Attoe C, et al: Simulation in psychiatry for medical doctors: a systematic review and meta-analysis. Med Educ 54(8):696–708, 2020 32242966

Rotenstein LS, Edwards ST, Landon BE: Adult primary care physician visits increasingly address mental health concerns. Health Aff (Millwood) 42(2):163–171, 2023 36745830

Satiani A, Niedermier J, Satiani B, Svendsen DP: Projected workforce of psychiatrists in the United States: a population analysis. Psychiatr Serv 69(6):710–713, 2018 29540118

Younes N, Delaunay AL, Roger M, et al: Evaluating the effectiveness of a single-day simulation-based program in psychiatry for medical students: a controlled study. BMC Med Educ 21(1):348, 2021 34134692

Part I

General Themes in Undergraduate Psychiatric Education

1

Integrating Psychological, Social, and Behavioral Concepts Into Undergraduate Medical Education

Lindsey S. Pershern, M.D.
Marika I. Wrzosek, M.D.

In this chapter, we explore priorities for incorporating psychological, social, and behavioral content in undergraduate medical education. These topic areas, which represent broad areas of science, are referred to by many terms; in this chapter, we use *psycho-social-behavioral.* We intend not to oversimplify these areas but rather to provide an easy "umbrella" term. In medical education, it is important to recognize and promote psycho-social-behavioral areas as theory-driven, hypothesis-based fields of study with value and importance in the practice of medicine.

We provide historical perspective on how behavioral science gained traction despite the traditional biomedical focus of medical education. We also present guidance on important topic areas for educators. There is consensus that physician understanding of psycho-social-behavioral topics improves patient care outcomes, health inequities, and individual professional development, but specific topics and educational methods vary widely (Association of American Medical Colleges 2011). We review topics relevant to medical educators, curriculum design priorities, and perspectives necessary to cultivate improved psycho-social-behavioral awareness in individual learners.

As holistically oriented clinicians in medical education systems, we are uniquely positioned to see the teaching potential in patients and their stories. Consider the parable of the blind men who tried to identify an elephant by each touching a different part. The physician who sees patients in a single context is like the blind man who insists he is touching a wall (the elephant's side), a rope (the tail), or a spear (the tusk). We want students, after learning relevant psycho-social-behavioral concepts, to recognize (or at least consider) the whole elephant.

History of Psycho-Social-Behavioral Concepts in Undergraduate Medical Education

The integration of psychological concepts into the medical school curriculum has a relatively modern history. Although Abraham Flexner did not initially include these concepts when crafting his 1910 report on medical education in the United States, he later revised recommendations to acknowledge the limitations of the heavy focus on the scientific method at the expense of social and humanistic content (Doukas et al. 2010). It took decades before medical education shifted from its "hard science" foundations to the inclusion of psychology and behavioral sciences. In the 1960s–1980s, medical schools were only starting to include behavioral science content in their curricula, with George Engel introducing the biopsychosocial model in 1977 (Carr 2017). During the 1990s and early 2000s, a new integrative model emerged that supplemented the biopsychosocial model to capture the interaction and integration of social, cultural, environmental, behavioral, and biological factors. By 2004, educators were promoting a broader perspective of the importance of behavioral and social science topics in medical education, culminating in the Institute of Medicine (IOM) report entitled "Improving Medical Education: Enhancing the Behavioral and Social Science Content of Medical School Curricula" (Cuff and Vaneslow 2004). The reasons for prioritizing these topics included the role of physicians in behavioral change and disease prevention, the importance of effective communication skills in relationships and within systems, and the need for self-reflection in the formation of a professional identity.

From theory to incorporation, modern medical schools rely on several key sources for their content priorities. Those outlined in the IOM report are listed in Table 1.1. Within each domain are important topics relevant to physician knowledge, perspectives, and skills. The Behavioral and Social Science Expert Panel of the Association of American Medical Colleges (AAMC) drew from these priorities to develop recommendations of essential foundations for future physicians (Association of American Medical Colleges 2011). In the review, they arrayed the IOM knowledge domains to each of six physician roles defined by the CanMEDS physician competency framework (Royal College of Physicians and Surgeons of Canada 2015) to create the Behavioral and Social Sciences Teaching Matrix. This tool guides educators in crafting specific educational activities to highlight relevant behavioral, psychological, and social domains. The content areas of the U.S. Medical Licensing Examination (USMLE) (Table 1.2) are a specific guide for medical educators.

Beyond the concrete applications of psychological concepts defined by IOM, AAMC, and USMLE, exposing students to behavioral science

Table 1.1 **Institute of Medicine Committee on Behavioral and Social Sciences in Medical School Curricula: behavioral and social science topic domains of high priority**

Mind–body interactions in health and disease
Patient behavior and behavior change
Physician role and behavior
Physician–patient interaction and communication
Social and cultural issues in health care
Health policy, economics, delivery (social factors)

Source. Adapted from Cuff and Vaneslow 2004.

Table 1.2 U S .Medical Licensing Examination Step 1 Content Outline: psychological, social, and behavioral topics

Human development	Normal age-related findings and care of the well patient Developmental stages: cognitive, psychosocial, anticipatory guidance Adaptive behavioral responses to stress and illness (e.g., coping mechanisms), patient adherence
Patient safety Strategies to reduce error	Teamwork: principles of highly effective teams; case management; physician teams, physician-physician communication; interprofessional/intraprofessional teams; strategies for communication among teams, including system-provider communication, interprofessional communication, provider-patient communication
Social sciences	Communication and interpersonal skills, including health literacy and numeracy and cultural competence Patient interviewing, consultation, and interactions with the family (patient-centered communication skills): • fostering the relationship (e.g., expressing interest) • information gathering (e.g., exploring patient's reaction to illness) • information provision (e.g., providing information about working diagnosis) • making decisions (e.g., eliciting patient's perspectives) • supporting emotions (e.g., effective discussion with difficult patients) • enabling patient behaviors (e.g., education and counseling)
Medical ethics and jurisprudence, including issues related to death and dying and palliative care	Physician–patient relationship (boundaries, confidentiality including HIPAA, privacy, truth-telling, and other principles of medical ethics, such as autonomy, justice, beneficence, and nonmaleficence)

Source. USMLE 2025.
HIPAA = Health Insurance Portability and Accountability Act.

content during their training prepares them to be the physicians we want in our medical systems and communities. Exposure to psycho-social-behavioral concepts is important for all students, and arguably even more important for those students who will not pursue a career in psychiatry. In their future roles as surgeons, obstetricians, oncologists, or primary care physicians, these students will benefit from the content and application of psychological concepts in their care of all patients in all practice settings. Their patients will also benefit from more psychologically aware physicians. In the preclinical curriculum, psychological, social, and behavioral education sets the stage for clinical experiences in clerkships. The priority in all basic science education is planting seeds that can sprout and come to life in the clinical context.

Teaching Methods/Pedagogy

As educators, you are likely thinking about how to incorporate these priorities into your course, rotation, mentorship, or advising relationship with students. Students may resist the presentation of psychological, social, and behavioral content because they question its relevance, perceive it as low value, or consider it too ideological or disconnected from the science. Educators must succeed in translating this content into the students' clinical experiences, as opposed to presenting abstractions and theories. To achieve this successfully, we suggest prioritizing methods that promote significance, engagement, reflection, and integration.

Promoting Significance for the Learner

The biomedical/medical causality model of traditional medical education can create a misalignment for students learning psychological, social, and behavior content. Cultivating the connection between these topics and their professional goals and identities as healers is crucial (Peterson et al. 2011). Strategies to increase significance in health professions education overlap with techniques in competency-based medical education, adaptive learning, and paradigm shifts (details of which are beyond the scope of this chapter). Drawing from that foundation, we can confidently assert that techniques to improve significance that draw the student into the domains proposed by Fink (2013) in "Creating Significant Learning Experiences" will benefit your course, class, or rotation. Fink defined the six domains as 1) foundational knowledge,

2) application, 3) integration, 4) learning how to learn (metacognition), 5) caring, and 6) the human dimension. With a lens to incorporate as many domains as possible, creating curricula provides opportunities for creativity and innovation that reward both educator and learner.

Taking an example from the USMLE outline, let's consider opportunities for enhancing significance. For the educator tasked with teaching about patient response to the diagnosis of ulcerative colitis, a foundational knowledge outline may include topics of development, coping, cultural factors, communication factors, and the impact of social determinants of health. Techniques for application and integration include exploration of a case of ulcerative colitis in an African American patient with a newly discovered genetic vulnerability, including delays in care due to economic, access, and education factors. As part of the activity, students can reflect and discuss their emotional reactions and potential biases. Revisiting the case during the gastrointestinal course or the medicine clerkship, perhaps pairing it with a session in which a patient living with ulcerative colitis conveys their personal experience, provides opportunities for integration that leverage the human dimension.

Educators should consider the educational psychology concepts of the zone of proximal development (ZPD) and scaffolding in curriculum design. The ZPD is the theoretical space between what a learner can do unassisted versus what they cannot do even if supported (Crain 2016). Scaffolding is the temporary help the educator provides as the student completes a learning task that would be difficult without such support (Masava et al. 2022). To build the necessary scaffold, a teacher may have to explicitly point out a concept in a way that will stick with the student.

Once engaged, students should be empowered. Students being able to take ownership and actively participate in patient care in a meaningful way is critically important as they develop professional identity (Wilson et al. 2013). When learners struggle to see their impact on a care team, we should reinforce that what they do matters. Some learners will be able to identify the impact they have; others will need some scaffolding. Be curious about what is interesting to the student, to help focus the clinical interaction on their learning goals. Arguably, this is most challenging when a student is "just" there on rotation for credit but does not feel invested. The educator may have to explicitly bridge interest and experience to provide a sufficient scaffold for student learning and retention. Even tapping into reflective questioning—"How do you think this may show up in [student's chosen field]?"—may stimulate this connection.

Promoting Engagement

Few medical student educators will need convincing that active learning modalities are preferred to traditional lectures; there is ample evidence of improved effectiveness (Freeman et al. 2014). The application of psychological, social, and behavioral concepts is especially important for preclinical learners. Before entering clerkships, students may not have personal experiences to draw from and connect to. For instance, they may not appreciate how family dynamics affect the advance directive planning of a patient with terminal disease. Innovative techniques discussed elsewhere in this book will be particularly useful for this content, including case-based, team-based, and problem-based learning (Chapter 15) and simulation (Chapter 17).

Narrative Medicine

The use of narrative in education aligns with the priorities of engagement, cultivation of empathy, and humanistic understanding in the medical context. This technique has been shown to promote empathy, reflection, professionalism, and trustworthiness in students. In addition, it improves communication and collaboration and fosters emotional support among colleagues. Descriptions of this technique include core elements of the three-step "read-reflect-respond" model (Fenstermacher et al. 2021). In this application, learners have opportunities to engage with a patient narrative through reflection, write about their personal experience of reflection, and discuss their reactions. Patient narratives can be drawn from a variety of sources, especially those in the humanities (art, literature, music, theater, and film).

Reflection

Reflection as a metacognitive process has been described in the medical education literature as critical for lifelong learning, developing professional expertise, and forging therapeutic relationships with patients (Sandars 2009). Early in their education, learners may need specific prompts to reflect on a certain aspect of their interaction with a patient or the health care team. Reflection is a tool (not a topic) that facilitates student learning. One of the most sought-after themes in medical education is a humanistic approach to patient care and the profession (Han et al. 2019). By promoting self-reflection, educators can facilitate the formation of learners' emerging professional identity.

Integration

Behavioral and social sciences courses that primarily stand alone or exist outside of the rest of the medical school content are at risk of being perceived as irrelevant to students. Integration is important to highlight relevance and application to the practice of medicine. Effective integration requires the consistent inclusion of psychological, social, and behavioral concepts in basic science courses, clinical courses, and nonpsychiatry clerkships. As psychiatric educators, we may not be in a position to make recommendations on the broader curriculum, but we can be present, collaborative, and conscientious of opportunities for integration to the benefit of the broader mission. The AAMC Behavioral and Social Sciences Foundations for Future Physicians is a good resource for integration strategies for leaders in undergraduate medical education (Association of American Medical Colleges 2011).

Cultivating Psychological Awareness in Medical Students Across Specialties

A curriculum, course, or learning session is successful if it has impact and reaches an individual learner with retention over time. As educators, we do not simply outline content—we serve as scaffolders, role models, and drivers of professional development. The domains from the IOM (Table 1.1) are omnipresent, cutting across all specialties. The USMLE content outline (Table 1.2) specifically includes normal processes within behavioral health that manifest across multiple patient interactions. Although learners pursuing psychiatry may be especially attuned to domains such as the mind–body interaction or social and cultural contexts, all learners need to be roughly aware of those domains and how they may affect patient care. Aside from instilling general rapport-building skills, you as educators can explicitly bring certain topics to learners' conscious awareness. What follows are themes and general topics that we recommend be instilled in medical students as part of training well-balanced physicians. Students who go into psychiatry will likely revisit these concepts while in training, but this may be the only exposure for those who pursue nonpsychiatric specialties.

The general thread is to think like a human first, physician second, and specialist third. We recognize that there are countless variations possible, and we present generalizable themes that educators can weave into their respective institution's curricular structure. We do not intend this to be an exhaustive or exclusive list.

Affect Tolerance and Labeling Feelings

Helping students find empathy for patients whose affects may be negative, strong, or otherwise unpleasant is something educators can do early and often. Most human beings respond with initial discomfort to people crying or being obviously distressed. Even toddlers are capable of empathy and may try to comfort someone they see as upset (Ornaghi et al. 2020). The ability to tolerate a patient's distress opens the door to learning more about its source.

Sometimes feelings manifest as behaviors. For instance, a patient who is banging on their gurney is likely feeling something. By being curious about these feelings and their triggers, the educator (together with the learner) can uncover a myriad of factors contributing to human behavior. Just as in psychotherapy, where therapists will sit with a patient's distress without necessarily alleviating it, so can medical students sit with patients and their distress as empathetic listeners, a crucial skill regardless of the setting. Modern medicine often underappreciates the skill of being able to sit with distress, a situation compounded by time pressure and an orientation to "fix problems." To not explore a distressed affect is akin to omitting a potentially painful, yet necessary, abdominal exam. Just as students are encouraged to be curious about patients' emotional states, so should educators be curious about their learners' experiences on the wards. When patients or students are "prickly," that is often a good time to lean in and find out more.

As students reflect, they may come face to face with uncomfortable feelings. It is critical that they perceive the learning environment as a safe space. It can be powerful to remind students that the entire range of feelings is normal, and that feelings are neither good nor bad. Some learners have a hard time identifying affective states, in themselves as well as in their patients. Educators should bear in mind the concept of displacement and the range of coping mechanisms patients and students may display. For instance, some students may resort to gallows humor (humor that "treats serious, frightening, or painful subject matter in a light or satirical way to address sadness or frustration" [Watson 2011]). By itself, such humor can be jarring, but it is not necessarily unethical. Acknowledging the range of emotions present on the wards—in treaters and patients alike—can lead to fruitful reflections and understanding of self. For example, you may have the opportunity to help a student understand that the patient who seems to be upset over something trivial, like their water not having ice, may really be displacing their fear, anger, or frustration. In a team situation, you may find that exploring a negative dynamic with the senior resident can lead to a fruitful discussion of bandwidth, burnout, and resilience.

Language and Stigma

Language used to describe patients can inadvertently propagate stigma and reinforce biases and health care disparities (Goddu et al. 2018). As learners present patients and plans, instructors will get glimpses of their assumptions. By reflecting on the language that students and the team use (such as "noncompliance," "difficult patient," or "refusing treatment"), educators can explore the meaning, intent, and impact of those words. They can model patient-first language ("the patient with alcohol use disorder" as opposed to "the alcoholic") in their interactions with students. Also, they can listen for descriptions based on temporary states ("the angry patient" describes an affect at a given moment, without much context) and correct them. Helping students bring to awareness the language they use, especially focusing on patient-centered language, is relevant across all specialties (Stagno et al. 2016).

Development

As students interact with patients, they will likely notice that people react differently to similar situations. Educators should ensure that students understand and consider the developmental stages of those with whom they interact. Erik Erikson described a series of eight life stages, cradle to grave, postulating that people have a certain task within each that they need to resolve (Crain 2016). Understanding someone's current life stage can help a student envision what to expect in the clinical encounter: a toddler will be more worried about if they can play after an injury than the long-term implications of injury, a 40-year-old may worry about picking up their kids from school if they are hospitalized, and an 80-year-old may be most concerned about the quality of their remaining life. Understanding developmental stages can also help learners appreciate perceived resistance to certain suggestions of the treatment team. Asking what is most important for the patient, coupled with an understanding of what is typical or expected at a given life stage, can yield discussions on care that are fruitful and not frustrating.

Development interacts with psychosocial forces. As important as patient autonomy is in clinical medicine, educators will be wise to remind students that autonomous patients do not exist in a vacuum, even if they are legally adults. Patients both affect and are affected by the people around them (e.g., their parents, children, friends, and other loved ones). For example, involving students in couple or family discussions presents an opportunity to illustrate that treatment recommendations exist in a context beyond the individual patient. When proposing interventions, students should consider the patient's situation and their values.

Students should be encouraged to consider developmental factors in clinical care. Examples of this are infinite; Table 1.3 lists some considerations according to life stage. If students internalize what is expected at each developmental stage, they will have the opportunity to recognize variations and target their communication accordingly. Educators also ought to display developmental awareness of their learners. Students experience their own developmental transitions that may spill over into how they approach patients or team members, and instructors may need to prioritize discussions to ensure the student is present and supported to engage in patient care.

Loss and Grief

Students will invariably encounter patients as they respond to loss. Grief response can be triggered not just by loss of life, but also by loss of health or function, representing the need to come to terms with reality as it is, not reality as previously envisioned. Educators can and should empower students to investigate what the illness has done to the patient's life (hopes, dreams, plans, identity). Part of sitting with distress is helping patients grieve the loss of "what might have been." For illustration, an athlete who underwent a traumatic amputation may struggle to accept their need for physical rehab; a parent whose child has suffered a traumatic brain injury may struggle to accept the need for special education resources. A treatment will be effective only if it has patient/family buy-in; understanding the patient's world helps highlight the priorities that need to align with treatment recommendations. Giving space for the patient and family to come to terms with their new reality is time well spent and fosters treatment collaboration.

Table 1.3 Patient developmental stage considerations

Developmental stage	Considerations for treater
Infant	• Infants may be nonverbal yet are still very communicative. • Parents will have concerns that need to be addressed before they consent to treatment.
Toddler	• Accept the child's growing autonomy. • Resist the urge to ask yes/no questions; instead offer no-choice choices ("Would you like me to look into your eyes or ears first?" instead of "Can I take a look at your ear?")
Preschool	• Engage the child in history-taking. • Make a point to ask about the child's fears and questions.
Latency (school-age)	• Feeling good and competent at something is important. • Ask the child and find that child's particular strength.
Adolescence	• Confidentiality is a frequent concern; emphasize honest boundaries of confidentiality ("I can keep what we discuss between us unless it involves your safety"). • Respect parental involvement even if parent and child disagree.
Young adulthood (20s and 30s)	• Recognize neurodevelopmental diversity (e.g. variations of levels of maturity in this age group). • Appreciate variable tolerance of risk and future consequences.
Mid-adulthood (40s–60s)	• Consider the roles and responsibilities that people are juggling (e.g., intimate partner, job, kids, aging parents). • Recognize that a likelihood of illness may impact future planning (e.g., a medical crisis draining savings).

Table 1.3 Patient developmental stage considerations *(continued)*

Developmental stage	Considerations for treater
Late adulthood (65+)	• Recognize the importance of end-of-life planning, ideally before acute crisis occurs. • Conversations should consider quality vs. simply quantity of life, and patients' wishes may vary from that of family members.

Conclusions

All specialties have a shared responsibility to incorporate psychological, social, and behavioral concepts during medical school. Holistically oriented clinicians, such as psychiatrists, psychologists, and other practitioners, can play a crucial role in emphasizing these concepts in curricular development through strategies that promote significance, engagement, reflection, and integration. When we break down psychological, social, and behavioral factors that affect patients' presentations, we address various aspects of the human condition that impact care: how people are built, how they deal with the world, and what the world has tossed to them. The focus on feelings and development may be uncomfortable for some students, so educators should foster a psychologically safe learning environment with a curious, nonjudgmental stance to facilitate growth and development. The more emphasis on psychological, social, and behavioral factors in patient care, the more likely our students will develop into the kind of doctors we would want to treat our loved ones.

Key Points

- Students should become aware of the impact that psychological, social, and behavioral factors have on patient care, regardless of the specialties they ultimately pursue.
- In designing curricula, educators should make a concerted effort to prioritize psychological, social, and behavioral concepts by incorporating teaching models that promote significance, foster engagement, and incorporate active learning and reflection

strategies while integrating these concepts across multiple clinical environments.

- When working with individual students, educators can elicit the psychological, social, and behavioral factors that may be relevant by bringing to awareness affect recognition, language use, developmental stages (of both patients and students), and people's response to loss and death.

References

Association of American Medical Colleges (AAMC): Behavioral and Social Science Foundations for Future Physicians. AAMC, 2011. Available at: https://www.aamc.org/media/31241/download. Accessed July 23, 2025.

Carr JE: The evolution of psychology as a basic bio-behavioral science in healthcare education. J Clin Psychol Med Settings 24(3–4):234–244, 2017 28825163

Crain W: Theories of Development: Concepts and Applications, 6th Edition. New York, Routledge, 2016

Cuff PA, Vaneslow NA: Improving Medical Education: Enhancing the Behavioral and Social Science Content of Medical School Curricula. Institute of Medicine Committee on Behavioral and Social Sciences in Medical School Curricula. Washington, DC, National Academies Press, 2004

Doukas DJ, McCullough LB, Wear S: Reforming medical education in ethics and humanities by finding common ground with Abraham Flexner. Acad Med 85(2):318–323, 2010 20107362

Fenstermacher E, Longley RM, Amonoo HL: Finding the story in medicine: the use of narrative techniques in psychiatry. Psychiatr Clin North Am 44(2):263–281, 2021 34049648

Fink LD: Creating Significant Learning Experiences; An Integrated Approach to Designing College Courses. San Francisco, CA, Wiley and Sons, 2013

Freeman S, Eddy SL, McDonough M, et al: Active learning increases student performance in science, engineering, and mathematics. Proc Natl Acad Sci U S A 111(23):8410–8415, 2014 24821756

Goddu AP, O'Conor KJ, Lanzkron S, et al: Do words matter? Stigmatizing language and the transmission of bias in the medical record. J Gen Intern Med 33(5):685–691, 2018 29374357

Han ER, Yeo S, Kim MJ, et al: Medical education trends for future physicians in the era of advanced technology and artificial intelligence: an integrative review. BMC Med Educ 19(1):460, 2019 31829208

Masava B, Nyoni CN, Botma Y: Scaffolding in health sciences education programmes: an integrative review. Med Sci Educ 33(1):255–273, 2022 37008420

Ornaghi V, Conte E, Grazzani I: Empathy in toddlers: the role of emotion regulation, language ability, and maternal emotion socialization style. Front Psychol 11:586862, 2020 33192920

Peterson CD, Rdesinski RE, Biagioli FE, et al: Medical student perceptions of a behavioural and social science curriculum. Ment Health Fam Med 8(4):215–226, 2011 23205062

Royal College of Physicians and Surgeons of Canada. CanMEDS Framework. Royal College of Physicians and Surgeons of Canada, 2015. Available at: https://www.royalcollege.ca/content/dam/document/standards-and-accreditation/2015-canmeds-framework-reduced-e.pdf. Accessed May 20, 2025.

Sandars J: The use of reflection in medical education: AMEE Guide No. 44. Med Teach 31(8):685–695, 2009 19811204

Stagno S, Crapanzano K, Schwartz A: Keeping the patient at the center: teaching about elements of patient-centered care. MedEdPORTAL 12:10500, 2016 30984842

United States Medical Licensing Exam (USMLE): USMLE® Content Outline (2025). Available at: https://www.usmle.org/sites/default/files/2022–01/USMLE_Content_Outline_0.pdf. Accessed July 23, 2025.

Watson K: Gallows humor in medicine. Hastings Cent Rep 41(5):37–45, 2011 21980898

Wilson I, Cowin LS, Johnson M, Young H: Professional identity in medical students: pedagogical challenges to medical education. Teach Learn Med 25(4):369–373, 2013 24112208

2

Mental Health and Well-Being in Medical Student Education

Stuart Slavin, M.D., M.Ed.

For about 20 years, there has been heightened concern about medical student well-being. A series of papers from researchers at the Mayo Clinic from 2006 to 2008 described a problematic mental health landscape. "Systematic Review of Depression, Anxiety, and Other Indicators of Psychological Distress Among U.S. and Canadian Medical Students" reviewed the broad mental health problems seen in medical students (Dyrbye et al. 2006a). The paper was followed by two multi-institutional studies that found burnout rates of 45% and 49.6% (Dyrbye et al. 2006b, 2008). In the second study, the rate of suicidal ideation for the previous year was 11.2%. More recently, a meta-analysis found a global rate of depression of 27.2% among medical students, a rate far higher than that of the general population. In the same study, the suicidal ideation rate was found to be 11.1% (Rotenstein et al. 2016).

Prompted in large part by these studies, medical schools across the United States have directed significant attention to the issue of mental health and well-being and instituted a range of well-being initiatives and programming. Given this, it is reasonable to ask whether there is evidence that these interventions are having a significant positive impact on students. The only national data set that is available to explore this question comes from surveys conducted by the Association of American Medical Colleges (AAMC). The Year Two Questionnaire (Y2Q) and the Graduation Questionnaire are surveys given to all medical students in the second year and the final year of medical school, respectively (Association of American Medical Colleges 2022a, 2022b). Although they do not contain questions related to depression and anxiety, they do assess elements of burnout as well as the medical school learning environment. Of significant concern is that these measures do not appear to be improving, and in some domains, they appear to be getting worse.

From 2016 to 2022, perceived stress, disengagement, exhaustion, emotional climate, quality of life, student–student interaction, and student–faculty interaction have all worsened; the decline in most of these measures preceded the pandemic (Association of American Medical Colleges 2022b) (see Table 2.1).

Results from the AAMC Graduation Questionnaire have not shown the level of decline seen in the Y2Q, but none of the burnout measures showed any improvement over the same 7-year span (Association of American Medical Colleges 2022a, 2022b) (see Table 2.2).

Interventions, at least at a national level, appear to be failing to have a measurable positive impact on student well-being. The reasons for the ineffectiveness of these collective interventions are not clear, but it may be that although the problem (like that facing practicing physicians)

Table 2.1 AAMC Year Two Questionnaire: stress, burnout, and emotional climate (mean scores)

Item	2016	2019	2021	2022
Perceived stress	5.7	6.0	6.1	6.1
Disengagement	9.7	10.0	10.4	10.2
Exhaustion	11.7	12.0	12.5	12.5
Emotional climate	9.2	9.1	8.8	9.1
Quality of life	40.6	40.3	38.9	39.5
Student–student interaction	14.9	14.7	13.7	14.7
Student–faculty interaction	14.7	14.7	14.2	14.4

Source. AAMC 2022b.

Table 2.2 AAMC Graduation Questionnaire: burnout and emotional climate (mean scores)

Item	2016	2019	2021	2022
Disengagement	9.8	9.9	9.7	9.8
Exhaustion	11.1	11.1	11.0	11.3
Emotional climate	9.7	9.7	9.6	9.6

Source. AAMC 2022a.

is largely environmental in nature, the vast majority of interventions are focused on individual strategies such as mindfulness, yoga, exercise, and healthy diets. These practices, although not unreasonable to encourage, do not address the root causes of the problem and are unlikely to be sufficient in solving it.

Guiding Principles for Action

When considering how to structure potential interventions to encourage well-being and positive mental health, some guiding principles can be informative.

- Understand the distinction between well-being and satisfaction. When well-being is the primary target, the result may be the kinds of interventions described above—positive steps and practices that can enhance well-being. An alternative target may be satisfaction—satisfaction with the experience of school, and also satisfaction with self, which is a struggle for many students. Focusing more on satisfaction might improve results.
- Individual strategies aren't all positive steps. It is important to help students develop skills to mitigate the negative impact of common problematic mindsets and automatic thoughts.
- Threats to mental health and well-being are primarily environmental in nature; thus most of the efforts should be directed at reducing or eliminating unnecessary stressors and enhancing the learning environment. We're not going to "resilience" our way out of this problem.
- Whenever possible, interventions should be guided by student perceptions of stressors, and students should be actively engaged in developing interventions.

- The goal for medical schools should be for their students to flourish, not just to reduce adverse mental health outcomes.
- Medical schools need to monitor the mental health and well-being of their students, ideally with (at least) annual surveys that include measures of depression, anxiety, and burnout. To these could also be added measures of flourishing, which are gaining prominence in the field. Without these assessments, schools will have no real idea whether their interventions are effective.

Environmental Interventions

The learning environment and associated threats to well-being in medical school vary dramatically depending on the phase of the curriculum. Three distinct phases—preclerkship, clerkship, and final year/application to residency—each pose unique threats to the well-being of students. I explore each of these phases below and then discuss individual threats to mental health.

Preclerkship Phase

Changes instituted over a 7-year period (2009–2015) at Saint Louis University School of Medicine serve as a model for change with the potential to enhance student well-being and decrease rates of depression and anxiety (Slavin 2019; Slavin and Chibnall 2016; Slavin et al. 2014). The initiatives were based on a simple model with three primary goals: 1) reduce or (when possible) eliminate unnecessary stressors and strive to enhance the learning environment; 2) provide students with the opportunity to develop skills to better manage stress; and 3) increase opportunities for students to find meaning in their work. The specific changes and years of implementation are listed in Table 2.3.

The impact on mental health outcomes was striking. Depression rates decreased by 85% in first-year students and 82% in second-year students compared with historical controls (prior to the interventions) (see Table 2.4).

First-year students' anxiety rates decreased by 75%, and those of second-years decreased by 47% (see Table 2.5). Of note, second-year students were surveyed at the end of the second curricular year, just as they embarked on their Step 1 studies, a fixed stressor that we could not change, and for which the experience of some degree of anticipatory anxiety might be viewed as a normal and appropriate reaction given the stakes involved.

Table 2.3 Well-being interventions in the preclerkship phase at Saint Louis University

Year	Interventions
2009	Pass/fail grading, 10% cut in curriculum time and curricular content, institution of longitudinal electives, theme-based learning communities
2010	2-hour resilience and mindfulness curriculum
2011	Changes to the position, structure, and grading practices of the Human Anatomy Course
2012	Change to "true" pass/fail grading (performance in the preclerkship phase not used to determine AOA eligibility and not shared with residency programs in the MSPE)
2014	Optional confidential tracking of depression and anxiety
2015	Focused academic and emotional support for second-year students in the run-up to USMLE Step 1

Source. Slavin 2019; Slavin and Chibnall 2016; Slavin et al. 2014.
AOA = Alpha Omega Alpha; MSPE = Medical Student Performance Evaluation; USMLE = U.S. Medical Licensing Examination.

The success of this initiative was grounded in and the result of a number of basic principles. The primary changes were environmental in nature, and these changes were guided in large part by students' perceptions of stressors and threats to their well-being. The changes were consistent with self-determination theory, in which individuals need to feel autonomy, competence, and relatedness to flourish. Students had

Table 2.4 Percentage of students with positive screens for depression

Graduating class	Orientation	M1 (end of year)	M2 (end of year)
2011	6	27	29
2012	6	27	35
2018	4	4	6

Source. Slavin 2019; Slavin and Chibnall 2016; Slavin et al. 2014.
M1 = first year of medical school; M2 = second year of medical school.

Table 2.5 Percentage of students with positive screens for anxiety

Graduating class	Orientation	MS1 (end of year)	M2 (end of year)
2011	33	56	58
2012	27	54	61
2018	21	14	32

Source. Adapted from Slavin and Chibnall 2016.
M1 = first year of medical school; M2 = second year of medical school.

substantial autonomy in choosing electives and other activities. They also had great autonomy in what and how much to study, rather than being motivated to study to chase scores and grades. Students who may have struggled in the core curriculum had new ways to feel competent through engagement in their electives and learning communities. Relatedness and relationships were also strengthened, not just between students, but also with faculty and community members, as students had new and greater opportunities to connect while engaged in their electives and their learning communities. That their experience was fundamentally different from student experience at other medical schools is borne out by results from the AAMC Y2Q (Table 2.6).

Strikingly, in the Y2Q survey, SLU students reported spending 1.5–2 hours less per day in class or studying, yet their Step 1 mean scores rose from 224 to 228, and their failure rate on the exam dropped from 4% to 2% from 2009 to 2015.

Clerkship Year

Challenges and threats to well-being are dramatically different in the clerkship year than in the preclerkship phase. Students are thrust into the clinical learning environment in an intensive way that many have not previously experienced. They become de facto members of health care teams, and their experiences are dramatically influenced by the faculty and residents (as well as nurses, allied health professionals, and patients themselves). Students may be exposed to death, suffering, and grief on the wards in ways they have not previously experienced. Students may also experience mistreatment at the hands of members of the health care team, and increasingly in recent years, from patients

Table 2.6 Year 2 questionnaire results: mean scores 2015

Item	National	Saint Louis University
Emotional climate	9.2	10.8
Quality of life	40.1	45.5
Perceived stress	5.8	4.7
Disengagement	9.7	8.2
Exhaustion	11.8	9.3

Source. Data from Association of American Medical Colleges 2022b.

and their families. Racial and ethnic minorities are especially targeted and experience micro- and macro-aggressions on a regular basis.

Hours spent in the clinical setting may be long on some clinical rotations, and students may have weekend duties and night call, so their discretionary time may feel extremely limited. In addition to their clinical hours and curricular time, students also have after-hours work that includes preparation for National Board of Medical Examiners (NBME) Subject Exams, other tests, and reading up on their patients. Because most medical schools continue to use grades in the clerkship year, students may face a culture of competition with each other that was not present in their preclerkship studies. Those with aspirations to enter highly competitive specialties are likely to feel even greater pressure to excel and obtain the highest grades possible. Finally, connections with fellow students may be negatively affected by this new competition for grades, the limited amount of discretionary time, and the physical distance and fragmentation of the class compared with the preclerkship phase as students rotate through a range of clinical sites.

While significant concern has rightly been raised about mistreatment and its impact on medical student mental health and well-being, there is some evidence that it may not be the greatest threat. In one study, three cohorts of students at the end of their clerkship year were asked to rate the extent of impact of 25 potential sources of demoralization (defined as undermining of confidence, determination, spirit, or morale) on a 5-point Likert scale (Slavin and Chibnall 2017). Strikingly, various forms of mistreatment were ranked the lowest. Mistreatment occurred—it just did not appear to have a profoundly negative impact on students in terms of causing demoralization. The highest rated factors were 1) working with unhappy residents, 2) working with unhappy faculty, 3) being ignored by residents, 4) feeling incompetent, 5) receiving an unfair evaluation by an attending, and 6) receiving an unfair evaluation by a resident.

The question is, given these various threats to well-being in the clerkship year, what interventions are most likely to enhance well-being? Residents and faculty determine the nature of the clinical learning environment, and efforts to improve their mental health and well-being are critically important. It is important to also note that some students, particularly those who are members of racial and ethnic minority groups, may be particular targets of exclusion and mistreatment, and efforts to ensure a fair, equitable, and supportive environment for all are essential. Efforts should also be directed at improving the accuracy and reliability of evaluations of students by residents and faculty, with special attention to remedying the potential for explicit and implicit bias in these evaluation systems. Reducing competition among students will likely be difficult, as it appears that most medical schools are (in many ways understandably) unwilling to move to pass/fail grading in the clerkship year.

Some potential interventions may be seen through the lens of self-determination theory. Students should be given some measure of autonomy where possible, for example, by allowing them to select specific clinical services on a particular clerkship. For instance, students who are interested in pediatrics may benefit from participating in a child psychiatry block. Clerkships should encourage different opportunities for students to demonstrate competence, not just with patient presentations on rounds but also by pursuing various topics and presenting to the team or in conferences. Finally, residents and faculty should work to develop strong relationships with students so that they feel like they are valued members of the clinical team.

Final Year and Application to Residency Phase

A primary stressor in the final year of medical school is the process of applying to residency programs. Understandably, students may feel significant worry and anxiety about whether they will be able to match into their desired specialty, in their desired programs and geographical locations. The sense of competition has increased markedly in recent years and the result, particularly in highly competitive specialties, is that students are often applying to dozens of residency programs. In 2022, for example, in orthopedic surgery, the average number of applications per U.S. M.D. or D.O. graduate was 90.0; that for otolaryngology was 80.6 (Association of American Medical Colleges 2023). Student Affairs offices are trying to encourage students to apply to fewer programs, but overall, these efforts have been largely unsuccessful. Of note, a program at the University of Chicago Pritzker School of Medicine Career that encourages adaptive behaviors in place of rules and guidelines has led to 30% fewer residency applications per student than the national average, without compromising match outcomes in any way (Woodruff et al. 2023).

Individual Interventions

A range of individual interventions and strategies are being encouraged at medical schools across the country. The most typical appear to be meditation, yoga, exercise, healthy eating, and encouraging adequate sleep. While these interventions are certainly reasonable to encourage, they are unlikely to solve the mental health crisis on their own. Environmental interventions are of primary importance; however, other individual interventions are also needed. Those that focus on helping students manage problematic mindsets and common cognitive distortions hold particular promise and were a centerpiece of the highly successful well-being initiative at Saint Louis University described earlier.

Many medical students enter medical school with long-standing mindsets and thought patterns that can contribute to their distress. The two most studied are impostor phenomenon and maladaptive perfectionism, which have both been found to correlate with depression and anxiety (Henning et al. 1998; Hu et al. 2019). Other problematic mindsets include

- performance as identity: feeling like you *are* a score or grade, that it is a measure of your value or worth, rather than you *got* a grade
- toxic comparison: feeling good about your performance only if you are outperforming others
- a fixed rather than a growth mindset: feeling like your abilities are set and cannot improve

These mindsets may be accompanied by a range of cognitive distortions including magnification, all-or-none thinking, overgeneralization, tunnel vision, catastrophization, and fortune-telling (predicting the future with certainty). These dysfunctional thought patterns may be associated with feelings or emotions of inadequacy, embarrassment, or shame, that themselves may correlate and potentially contribute to depression and anxiety symptoms.

Students can be taught to manage and combat these thought patterns through simple-to-teach cognitive restructuring techniques. Cognitive restructuring forms the basis of cognitive-behavioral therapy, which remains a common treatment modality for anxiety and depression; these techniques can also be taught in a preventive fashion to groups. Cognitive restructuring was the centerpiece of the Saint Louis University resilience program. It can also be taught in small groups or supported by online apps.

Access to Mental Health Care

Given the high rates of depression and anxiety in medical students, ready access to high-quality mental health care is critically important. Ideally these services should be free or low cost and should be delivered by therapists who are familiar with the threats to mental health that students face. Access to care by itself is not sufficient. Also needed are efforts to reduce stigma and promote care-seeking through peer support programs, as well as teaching students and faculty psychological first aid techniques.

Conclusions

Despite significant attention to medical student mental health and well-being in recent years, the problem appears to continue unabated. New interventions are needed to address this problem, which will, hopefully, lead to a new era in medical education in which students experience a learning environment and curricular experiences that promote well-being rather than threaten it.

Key Points

- Over the past two decades, there have been ongoing concerns about the mental health and well-being of medical students.
- Even though medical schools across the United States have instituted a range of well-being initiatives and programming aiming

at addressing these concerns, the impact of such initiatives at a national level has been limited, as most of them focus on individual coping strategies and not on the primary threats to mental health and well-being among medical students, which seem largely environmental in nature.

- Interventions targeting environmental factors need to take into consideration the different phases of medical school training (preclerkship, clerkship, and final year/application to residency) as each one of them offers unique threats to the well-being of students.
- The availability of high-quality mental health care, free or at low cost and delivered by therapists familiar with the threats to mental health faced by medical students, is essential.

References

Association of American Medical Colleges (AAMC): Medical School Graduation Questionnaire All Schools Reports. AAMC, 2022a. Available at: https://www.aamc.org/data-reports/students-residents/report/graduation-questionnaire-gq. Accessed September 17, 2023.

Association of American Medical Colleges (AAMC): Medical School Year Two Questionnaire All Schools Reports. AAMC, 2022b. Available at: https://www.aamc.org/data-reports/students-residents/report/year-two-questionnaire-y2q. Accessed September 17, 2023.

Association of American Medical Colleges (AAMC): ERAS Statistics 2023. AAMC, 2023. Available at: https://www.aamc.org/data-reports/data/eras-statistics-data-2023. Accessed September 27, 2023.

Dyrbye LN, Thomas MR, Shanafelt TD: Systematic review of depression, anxiety, and other indicators of psychological distress among U.S. and Canadian medical students. Acad Med 81(4):354–373, 2006a 16565188

Dyrbye LN, Thomas MR, Huntington JL, et al: Personal life events and medical student burnout: a multicenter study. Acad Med 81(4):374–384, 2006b 16565189

Dyrbye LN, Thomas MR, Massie FS, et al: Burnout and suicidal ideation among U.S. medical students. Ann Intern Med 149(5):334–341, 2008 18765703

Henning K, Ey S, Shaw D: Perfectionism, the impostor phenomenon and psychological adjustment in medical, dental, nursing and pharmacy students. Med Educ Sep;32(5):456–464, 1998

Hu KS, Chibnall JT, Slavin SJ: Maladaptive perfectionism, impostorism, and cognitive distortions: threats to the mental health of pre-clinical medical students. Acad Psychiatry 43:381–385, 2019

Rotenstein LS, Ramos MA, Torre M, et al: Prevalence of depression, depressive symptoms, and suicidal ideation among medical students: a systematic review and meta-analysis. JAMA 316(21):2214–2236, 2016 27923088

Slavin S: Reflections on a decade leading a medical student well-being initiative. Acad Med 94(6):771–774, 2019 30489287

Slavin SJ, Chibnall JT: Finding the why, changing the how: improving the mental health of medical students, residents, and physicians. Acad Med 91(9):1194–1196, 2016 27166866

Slavin SJ, Chibnall JT: Mistreatment of medical students in the third year may not be the problem. Med Teach 39(8):891–893, 2017 28097902

Slavin SJ, Schindler DL, Chibnall JT: Medical student mental health 3.0: improving student wellness through curricular changes. Acad Med 89(4):573–577, 2014 24556765

Woodruff JN, Lee WW, Vela M, Davidson AI: Beyond compliance: growth as the guiding value in undergraduate medical education. Acad Med 98(6):S39–S45, 2023

3

Stigma and Attitudes Toward Psychiatry Among Medical Students: A Case Study

Khalid Bazaid, M.D.
Abdellah Bezzahou, M.D.

The escalating demand for mental health services underscores the indispensable role of psychiatry in modern health care. This trend exists against a backdrop of a global shortage of psychiatrists, which is exacerbated by the enduring stigma surrounding mental health that also significantly influences the field's perception among medical students. This situation poses a complex challenge: how do we inspire the next generation of medical professionals to pursue psychiatry, thereby mitigating the profound shortage of mental health practitioners? Notably, the chronic psychiatrist shortage in regions such as Ontario, Canada, vividly illustrates this dilemma, contributing to a broader mental health crisis that demands innovative solutions (Coalition of Ontario Psychiatrists 2018).

The critical intersection of medical education and psychiatric workforce development presents an opportunity to reshape students' perceptions and career trajectories. Clerkship rotations in psychiatry are particularly pivotal, offering direct exposure to the psychiatric field, which, according to some studies, can potentially diminish stigma and foster a more positive outlook toward the discipline (Lyons 2014). The literature presents a dichotomy of outcomes, with some findings suggesting that these educational experiences significantly influence students' attitudes and career decisions toward psychiatry (Lyons 2014) and others indicating a more nuanced impact, not always resulting in increased interest in the specialty (Das and Chandrasena 1988).

The stigma associated with psychiatry extends beyond patient care, permeating medical education and influencing students' attitudes toward the specialty. This stigma, characterized by enduring misconceptions and biases against mental illness and psychiatric treatment, remains a formidable barrier to attracting new entrants into the field (Walters et al. 2007). Medical students' attitudes toward psychiatry are a critical indicator of the field's future, as positive perceptions increase the likelihood of choosing psychiatry as a career path (Farooq et al. 2014).

In this context, we examine the results of a study we conducted at the University of Ottawa (unpublished) to exemplify and critically examine the influence of educational experiences, specifically psychiatry clerkship rotations, on medical students' attitudes toward psychiatry. The study, conducted during the 2020–2021 academic year, assessed the shift in attitudes among medical students before and after their psychiatry clerkship, thereby providing invaluable insights into the potential of clerkships to alter perceptions and encourage students toward a career in psychiatry. This examination is crucial for devising strategies to enhance the appeal of psychiatry as a profession, addressing the acute shortage of psychiatrists amid an escalating mental health crisis.

Expanding Horizons: Understanding Medical Students' Attitudes Toward Psychiatry

The burgeoning field of psychiatry inhabits an ever-evolving healthcare landscape, contending with global challenges of mental health crises and the pervasive stigma associated with mental disorders. A critical factor in navigating these challenges is understanding and influencing the attitudes of medical students toward psychiatry, as these perceptions significantly shape the future of mental health care.

This brief review delves into the nuanced factors influencing these attitudes, synthesizing insights from recent scientific literature.

Educational Exposure and Clinical Rotations

The impact of educational exposure on medical students' attitudes toward psychiatry is profound. Clinical rotations in psychiatry are pivotal, providing students with firsthand exposure to the field and directly influencing their perceptions and career choices. The research underscores the role of these rotations in demystifying psychiatric practice and fostering a more positive outlook toward the discipline. Lyons (2014) highlighted the transformative potential of direct clinical exposure in reducing stigma and enhancing students' appreciation of psychiatry as a viable career path. The curriculum's structure and content, as well as educators' attitudes, significantly shape students' perspectives, suggesting that a well-designed psychiatric curriculum is paramount in cultivating a positive outlook toward the field.

Stigma and Mental Health Literacy

Systemic and social stigma significantly influences medical students' attitudes toward psychiatry. The perpetuation of stereotypes and misconceptions about mental illness and psychiatric treatment within and outside the medical community deters interest in psychiatry. Educational initiatives aimed at improving mental health literacy can mitigate these effects by providing accurate information, challenging stereotypes, and highlighting the critical role of psychiatrists in health care. Programs that encourage empathy, understanding, and respect for individuals with mental health conditions can transform perceptions and foster a more inclusive and compassionate view of psychiatry.

Cultural and Personal Factors

The cultural background of medical students plays a crucial role in shaping their attitudes toward psychiatry. Cultural beliefs about mental health and illness, familial attitudes, and societal norms can facilitate or hinder students' openness to psychiatry. Al-Imam et al. (2024) explored how cultural divergence in psychedelic use among medical students offers insights into broader cultural influences on attitudes toward psychiatric practices. Additionally, factors such as resilience, gratitude, and personal experiences with mental health significantly affect students' perceptions. As Hahn et al. (2024) suggested, fostering resilience and gratitude could positively influence students' mental health and attitudes toward the psychiatric field.

Career Considerations and Role Models

Career considerations, including perceived prestige, financial incentives, and job security, influence the decision to pursue psychiatry. The availability of role models in psychiatry—mentors who exemplify the profession's values, skills, and satisfaction—can significantly sway students' career choices. Exposure to enthusiastic and dedicated psychiatric professionals during educational and clinical experiences can inspire students and challenge preconceived notions about the field.

Impact of Research Opportunities

Engagement in psychiatric research offers another avenue to positively influence students' attitudes toward psychiatry. Participation in research fosters an understanding of the complexities and challenges within the field, encouraging a more nuanced and informed perspective. Research opportunities allow students to contribute to advancing psychiatric knowledge, potentially sparking a lifelong interest in the field.

University of Ottawa Study

We conducted a study, "Impact of Psychiatry Clerkship Rotation on Medical Student Attitudes Toward Psychiatry at the University of Ottawa: A Pre and Post Survey," that serves as a reference point for our discussion on enhancing medical students' attitudes toward psychiatry. The study's primary objective was to evaluate how medical students' attitudes toward psychiatry changed following their clerkship experience. By understanding these shifts in attitudes, the study aimed to identify factors that could potentially enhance interest in psychiatry as a career among medical students.

Ninety-seven medical students at the University of Ottawa participated in this quasi-experimental study, providing a response rate of approximately 48%. The ATP-30 measure (Attitudes Toward Psychiatry-30 items), a validated tool developed by Burra et al. (1982)

to provide a comprehensive overview of attitudes toward the field, was used to evaluate students' attitudes before and after their psychiatry clerkship rotation. ATP-30 encompasses a range of factors, from the perceived efficacy of psychiatric treatment to the societal stigma associated with mental health disorders.

In our study, ATP-30 revealed significant improvements in students' attitudes toward psychiatry post-clerkship. Notably, the dimensions that showed the most marked positive change were those related to the perceived effectiveness of psychiatric treatments and the importance of psychiatry within the broader medical field. This shift suggests that direct exposure to psychiatric practice not only enhances students' understanding of psychiatric disorders and their treatments but also elevates the perceived status of psychiatry as a critical medical specialty.

The positive correlation between psychiatric clerkship rotations and improved attitudes toward psychiatry suggests that these educational experiences are crucial in shaping students' perspectives. This correlation is particularly relevant in addressing the ongoing challenges in psychiatrist recruitment and the broader mental health service demands. By providing students with direct exposure to psychiatric practice, these rotations can play a significant role in enhancing interest in the field, addressing misconceptions, and potentially contributing to the recruitment of future psychiatrists.

Other Research on the Role of Psychiatry Clerkships for Reducing Stigma

Other studies have shown a notable improvement in students' attitudes toward psychiatry post-clerkship, highlighting the effectiveness of direct exposure to psychiatric practice in demystifying the field and enhancing its appeal as a viable career path (Lyons and Janca 2015; Xavier et al. 2010). Studies have demonstrated significant improvements in students' interest in, knowledge of, and consideration of psychiatry as a career following clerkship experiences (Lyons and Janca 2015). These findings corroborate that well-structured psychiatric clerkships can positively influence medical students' career choices, contributing to a more robust psychiatric workforce.

The extent of these changes can vary, however, highlighting the importance of context, curriculum design, and the quality of the clerkship experience (Amsalem et al. 2020). Most studies reported positive shifts in attitudes toward psychiatry, but the degree of change and the aspects most influenced differed. For example, one study found improvements in students' comfort with psychiatric patients and an increased recognition of psychiatry's scientific basis post-clerkship (Xavier et al. 2010). These variances underscore the multifaceted impact of psychiatric education and the need for ongoing evaluation to optimize clerkship experiences.

The generalizability of findings across different educational and cultural contexts remains a challenge, as does the need for longitudinal data to assess the long-term impact of clerkship experiences on career choices in psychiatry. Future research should address these limitations by incorporating diverse study populations and longitudinal designs and examining the specific components of clerkships that contribute most significantly to changing attitudes toward psychiatry (Lyons and Janca 2015; Xavier et al. 2010). Moreover, exploring interventions targeted at reducing stigma and enhancing empathy toward psychiatric patients within the clerkship curriculum could offer additional insights into optimizing medical education in psychiatry (Amsalem et al. 2020). Such interventions, including direct patient contact and small-group discussions, have shown promise in reducing stigma and improving attitudes toward psychiatry among medical students.

Conclusions

Psychiatric clerkships represent a critical juncture in medical education, offering a unique opportunity to influence future health care professionals' attitudes toward psychiatry. By fostering positive perceptions, reducing stigma, and enhancing understanding of psychiatric practice, these educational experiences can contribute significantly to addressing the psychiatrist shortage and improving mental health care delivery. Ongoing research and innovation in medical education are essential to maximize the potential of psychiatric clerkships in shaping the next generation of psychiatrists.

The collective body of research emphasizes the significant influence of psychiatric clerkship rotations on medical students' attitudes toward psychiatry. Studies have consistently shown that psychiatric clerkships can lead to improved attitudes toward psychiatry, increased interest in the field, and a deeper understanding of psychiatric illnesses and their treatments. For instance, the positive shifts in student perceptions post-clerkship rotations highlight the clerkships' effectiveness in demystifying psychiatric practice and fostering a more positive outlook toward the field (Lyons and Janca 2015; Xavier et al. 2010). The introduction of direct patient contact and educational interventions targeting stigma reduction has been proven effective in enhancing empathy and reducing stigma toward mental illness among medical students (Amsalem et al. 2020). These findings hold profound implications for medical education and the future of psychiatry, suggesting that carefully designed clerkship rotations, supplemented with targeted anti-stigma interventions, can significantly contribute to cultivating a robust and empathetic psychiatric workforce.

Call to Action

In light of these findings, educational policymakers and medical schools must recognize and harness the critical role of psychiatric clerkship rotations in shaping medical students' attitudes and career choices. The evidence points to the need for integrating comprehensive, experiential learning opportunities that not only provide medical students with exposure to psychiatric practice but also actively work toward dispelling myths and reducing the stigma associated with mental health conditions.

To this end, medical schools should endeavor to

1. Ensure that psychiatric clerkships offer a well-rounded experience, including exposure to various psychiatric conditions and treatment modalities.
2. Incorporate anti-stigma programs and empathy-building exercises into the clerkship curriculum to foster positive attitudes toward patients with mental illness.
3. Facilitate opportunities for mentorship with psychiatry professionals to provide students with role models and career guidance.
4. Conduct ongoing research to identify the most effective components of psychiatric clerkships and refine them to maximize their impact on student attitudes.

The current psychiatrist shortage poses a significant challenge to mental health care delivery worldwide. Addressing this issue requires a concerted effort to make psychiatry an attractive and fulfilling career choice for future generations of medical professionals. The clerkship rotation in psychiatry emerges as a pivotal educational intervention in this effort, capable of transforming student perceptions and encouraging more students to enter the field of psychiatry.

Educational policymakers and medical schools are thus called on to prioritize the enhancement of psychiatric clerkship rotations, leveraging them as a strategic tool not only for educational enrichment but also as a means to bolster the psychiatric workforce. By doing so, we can hope to make significant strides toward a future where access to comprehensive, compassionate psychiatric care is a reality for all those in need.

Key Points

- Psychiatric clerkships can positively affect students' attitudes toward psychiatry and mental disorders.
- Direct contact with patients and educational interventions targeting stigma reduction during the psychiatric clerkship are effective in increasing empathy and reducing stigma toward mental illness.
- Schools should strive to offer carefully designed clerkship rotations and anti-stigma interventions, given the profound implications they can have toward cultivating a robust and empathetic psychiatric workforce.

References

Al-Imam A, Motyka MA, Michalak L: Cultural divergence in psychedelic use among medical students: an ESPAD-adapted survey among Poles and Iraqis. Eur J Investig Health Psychol Educ 14(3):563–583, 2024 38534899

Amsalem D, Gothelf D, Dorman A, et al: Reducing stigma toward psychiatry among medical students: a multicenter controlled trial. Prim Care Companion CNS Disord 22(2):19m02527, 2020

Burra P, Kalin R, Leichner P, et al: The ATP 30: a scale for measuring medical students' attitudes to psychiatry. Med Educ 16(1):31–38, 1982 7057722

Coalition of Ontario Psychiatrists: Ontario Needs Psychiatrists: Chronic Psychiatry Shortage Contributing to Canada's Mental Health Crisis. Ontario Psychiatric Association, 2018. Available at: https://www.cacap-acpea.org/wp-content/uploads/Ontario-Needs-Psychiatrists.pdf. Accessed May 15, 2024.

Das MP, Chandrasena RD: Medical students' attitude towards psychiatry. Can J Psychiatry 33(9):783–787, 1988

Farooq K, Lydall GJ, Malik A, et al: Why medical students choose psychiatry: a 20 country cross-sectional survey. BMC Med Educ 14(12), 2014

Hahn R, Brzoska P, Kiessling C: On the correlation between gratitude and resilience in medical students. GMS J Med Educ 41(1):Doc8, 2024

Lyons Z: Impact of the psychiatry clerkship on medical student attitudes towards psychiatry and to psychiatry as a career. Acad Psychiatry 38(1):35–42, 2014 24464416

Lyons Z, Janca A: Impact of a psychiatry clerkship on stigma, attitudes towards psychiatry, and psychiatry as a career choice. BMC Med Educ 15(34), 2015

Walters K, Raven P, Rosenthal J, et al: Teaching undergraduate psychiatry in primary care: the impact on student learning and attitudes. Med Educ 41(1):100, 2007

Xavier M, Almeida JC, Almeida SA: Impact of clerkship in the attitudes toward psychiatry and among Portuguese medical students. BMC Med Educ 10:56, 2010 20678213

4

Fostering Interest in Psychiatry Among Medical Students

Gabriella M. Thiessen, M.D.
J. Chase Findley, M.D.

Selecting a specialty for residency training is one of the most consequential events in the professional life of a physician. Choosing the specialty that best aligns with one's unique characteristics is critical in realizing one's potential to provide excellent patient care and find career fulfillment. It is therefore critical that the faculty of a medical school are committed to providing the opportunities and guidance necessary to assist future physicians in finding their ideal space within the medical profession.

Multiple factors—such as geographic distribution of residency programs, number of available positions, and funding issues—influence the distribution of physicians after graduation from medical school, but student preference ultimately has the greatest impact in shaping the future workforce for each specialty. The capability of the field of psychiatry to provide for the growing mental health needs of the community and to advance scientific understanding of mental illness is thus contingent on fostering student interest in psychiatry on a continuous basis. In this chapter, we provide an overview of the opportunities within a medical school to ensure that psychiatry attracts a plentiful and diverse group of future physicians who are likely to find personal satisfaction and professional success within our specialty.

Myriad internal and external factors influence student interest in the many specialties and subspecialties encountered during training. Some (such as temperament, personal values, and familial expectations) are intrinsic to individual students and are already present at matriculation to medical school. Others (such as the structure of the psychiatry clerkship or the availability of psychiatry-related extracurricular activities) are within faculty control and vary between institutions (Querido et al. 2016). The medical school that students attend can greatly increase or decrease students' interest in a given specialty, and schools should pay close attention to how a positive student experience of psychiatry is promoted through espoused faculty values, institutional culture, and curriculum structure (Spollen et al. 2017).

Students' specialty interests are not fixed but rather develop over the course of training, as shown by research that only a minority of students accurately anticipate their future specialty choice at the beginning of medical school. One study found that 80% of eventual psychiatry residents did not anticipate applying to psychiatry residency at matriculation, illustrating the dramatic potential for change in students' interests through medical training and the capability for impactful experiences in psychiatry to change students' career plans (Goldenberg et al. 2017). Interest in psychiatry tends to increase throughout medical school. Research has also found that students who enter medical school with an interest in psychiatry are more likely than those interested in other specialties to maintain their specialty interest until graduation, which underlines the importance of early identification and nurturing of students with an early predilection toward psychiatry.

Faculty involved in student education are working during an exciting era in the history of the specialty. Interest in psychiatry peaked following World War II, in part due to societal recognition of the mental health impacts of wartime trauma, after which the number of students applying to psychiatry declined and remained low from the 1970s until the early 2010s (Wilbanks et al. 2017). Encouragingly, psychiatry has markedly grown in popularity over the past decade, with an increasing number of students applying to the specialty each year. Factors leading to this change may involve shifting generational career priorities, decreasing focus on prestige and compensation, increasing focus on lifestyle factors, evolving attitudes about mental health care, and emerging destigmatization of mental illness (Russo et al. 2020). Although this trend is reassuring, societal need for mental health care continues to outpace the supply of new psychiatrists, and it must not be assumed that student interest in psychiatry will remain high without continued faculty effort. Faculty must strive to continue cultivating an educational experience that facilitates robust recruitment to our specialty.

High School and Undergraduate Education Years

Medicine is widely considered an art as well as a science. This may be particularly true of our specialty, which exists at the beautifully complex intersections of neuroscience, psychology, and social context (Kumar 2014). The dual commitment to science and to the human condition is reflected in the vibrant mosaic of psychiatrists whose educational paths, life experiences, and career aspirations often color outside the lines of the traditional premedical prescription.

The desire to pursue medicine is often sparked in the formative high school and undergraduate years. For many budding psychiatrists, these years contain catalysts that encourage them on their path toward psychiatry. Whether they witness a loved one's struggles with mental health or stumble on a captivating psychology course, students' experiences may be profound enough to kindle a lasting curiosity, if not a lifelong vocation.

Several underlying factors in the high school and undergraduate years are associated with choosing psychiatry as opposed to other medical specialties. Medical students who graduated from college with a psychology major or a bachelor of arts degree (B.A.) are more likely to specialize in psychiatry than their peers (Goldenberg et al. 2017). A number of other factors have been linked to choosing psychiatry, including having a mother who is a physician, taking undergraduate English literature and psychology electives for enjoyment, beginning medical school after the age of 27, and having substantial interaction with the LGBTQ+ community before medical school (Goldenberg et al. 2017). When medical school admissions committees are aware of these factors, they can be intentional in admitting students with an underlying inclination or aptitude for psychiatry. Psychiatry faculty members should participate in admissions committees and should recruit students into medical school who are likely to specialize in psychiatry. Additionally, premedical offices at undergraduate institutions should be deliberate about promoting medical school to psychology majors.

A shift toward a multidisciplinary approach to medicine has become increasingly pronounced in recent years, most evidently in 2015 when the Association of American Medical Colleges launched a new version of the Medical College Admissions Test (MCAT). Grounded in the belief that science alone is insufficient preparation for the practice of modern medicine, the 2015 MCAT introduced a section called the Psychological, Social, and Biological Foundations of Behavior. The addition makes up a quarter of the exam and requires students to apply scientific reasoning to the social and behavioral sciences. Covering psychology, sociology, biology, biochemistry, chemistry, physics, critical analysis, and reasoning, the updated MCAT makes medical school more accessible to the kind of students who are likely to apply to psychiatry and invites these students to showcase their multidisciplinary skillset.

Preclinical Medical School Years

The preclinical curriculum is likely the first inflection point in a student's path to becoming a psychiatrist. Although many students matriculate with some knowledge of mental health topics through personal experiences or prior coursework, the preclinical curriculum will be the first formal experience with psychiatric diagnoses and treatments for the majority of students. Some students, such as psychology majors or those with mental health professionals in their family, may have developed a positive impression of the specialty. Others may hold negative biases about mental health disorders due to the influence of media, family and friends, or many other sources. The preclinical course director is thus faced with the challenge of stimulating the interest of students already positively oriented toward psychiatry alongside those who may be disinterested or biased against the specialty. All the while, the preclinical course director must ensure the primacy of students learning the information necessary for patient care on clerkships and licensing examinations.

The majority of medical schools use a systems-based curriculum in which psychiatry content is delivered in a neuroscience-focused course. Such courses are often codirected with faculty from departments of neuroscience or neurology and integrate basic science disciplines including pharmacology, biochemistry, and pathology. With the multidisciplinary and voluminous nature of material presented during these courses, it is imperative that psychiatry faculty assume a prominent role in student-facing course leadership—ideally as a course director or codirector—and advocate for thorough representation of psychiatry content. Students will likely build their first impression of the profession of psychiatry from the preclinical course director and the clinical faculty teaching the course; thus the reputation of these faculty among students is of great importance. The course director should recruit faculty who demonstrate enthusiasm for psychiatry and are capable of delivering entertaining and effective sessions. These faculty members should have a positive attitude toward students and be receptive to student feedback.

Students value establishing connections between preclinical coursework and their future care of patients, which is best provided by clinicians practicing in the content area of their sessions. Faculty should be encouraged to emphasize the clinical aspects of their material: sharing illustrative patient anecdotes, highlighting stories of successful holistic treatment of patients, and describing the fulfillment that comes from practicing psychiatry and advocating for patients living with mental illness. Faculty should emphasize the medical basis for psychiatry and provide horizontal curriculum integration with other preclinical content, such as endocrine or autoimmune disorders.

The role of psychiatry faculty is not limited to a single course in a preclinical curriculum. Rather, opportunities for positively representing the specialty may be found in other courses such as those focused on physical examination and history-taking skills, or in other curricular components such as problem-based learning, professionalism seminars, and other small-group sessions. Psychiatry faculty should be encouraged to volunteer for these opportunities to both provide a psychiatric perspective on the curriculum content and demonstrate that psychiatrists are integral members of the medical education community. In addition, by engaging in any preclinical activities, faculty may develop student connections through which they can individually encourage students to consider psychiatry as a career and offer opportunities for further learning, such as shadowing, case reports, or research projects. Such early and repeated exposure to psychiatry in multiple venues, including both required and elective opportunities, may have a significant impact in stimulating early interest in psychiatry during the preclinical years (Holt et al. 2019).

Psychiatry Clerkship

The clerkship is the most important curriculum component for developing student interest in psychiatry (Crowley et al. 2023; Kim et al. 2023), and psychiatry departments seeking to recruit students must be willing to contribute considerable resources to providing a high-quality experience. Student perceptions of psychiatry often improve as a result of their clerkship experiences (Lyons 2014), and high student ratings of clerkship quality are associated with selection of psychiatry for residency training (Goldenberg et al. 2017). As longer clerkship length is associated with psychiatry career selection, psychiatry departments should advocate for equitable distribution of clerkship time with other departments, which may require discussions between the chairperson and dean's office.

The clerkship director plays a critical role in recruitment while also having the primary responsibility of providing the only clinical education in psychiatry for the vast majority of students who will not enter psychiatry residency. To accomplish these responsibilities, the clerkship director must be allotted adequate protected time, sponsored by either the department or the medical school. Like the preclinical course director, the clerkship director should be a highly reputable and inspirational physician who is able to appeal to students, adapt to evolving educational best practices, and engage in continuous educational quality improvement. The clerkship director must be readily accessible to students and serve as a strong advocate for student interests in interactions with departmental and health system leadership. The clerkship director should curate a selection of rich clinical experiences emphasizing the diversity of psychiatric diagnoses and treatments along with impactful didactic sessions, including the use of simulations and other active learning modalities. As students are highly attuned to the quality of the organization and administration of the course, the clerkship director must partner with a capable clerkship coordinator to meet logistical expectations such as rotation scheduling, distribution of evaluation and feedback forms, and prompt submission of grades (Russo et al. 2021).

Providing students with exposure to subspecialties, particularly child-adolescent psychiatry, may provide opportunities to capture interest in psychiatry from students who may be also considering other specialties such as pediatrics. The clerkship should have elective learning opportunities for interested students, which may include brief assignments to other services apart from their primary rotation, psychotherapy group sessions, observation of interventional psychiatry treatments, or attendance at resident conferences. Students showing an interest in psychiatry or demonstrating advanced patient care skills related to psychiatry should be identified and encouraged to take advantage of such opportunities.

Student interactions with residents play an important role in specialty choice, and clerkships with associated residency programs should facilitate interactions between students and residents. Studies have shown that the reputation of residents within a specialty influences student specialty choice, and residents should thus be equipped to provide excellent supervision and teaching of students. Students may be influenced by their "near-peer" learner relationship to residents when considering specialty options and be better able to visualize their future selves in the role of resident as compared with faculty. Interventions to develop residents as educators may include organizing didactic workshops focused on teaching skills, providing feedback to residents on their teaching performance from student evaluations, appointing a chief resident of student education, and presenting an annual student education award.

Senior Electives

Senior electives bridge the daunting gap between medical student and resident. The framework built into the fourth year of medical school should ideally offer flexibility for students to finalize their choice of specialty, apply to residency programs, prepare for intern-level responsibilities, and nurture specific areas of interest. Whereas third-year clerkships usually rule specialties in or out for a particular student, fourth-year electives largely confirm a student's existing career aspirations. The psychiatry department should offer an array of senior electives to meet the needs of psychiatry applicants as well as students still choosing between specialties.

The number of psychiatry residency applications and the number of positions filled continue to increase every year. With an impressive fill rate of 99%, the 2,164 psychiatry residency positions available in 2023 represented the highest number of offerings in our specialty to date (National Resident Matching Program 2023). As the number of psychiatry residency applicants continues to climb, medical schools should mirror this increased demand with an ample, diverse supply of psychiatry electives for fourth-year students.

Quite unlike any other aspect of medicine, psychotherapy can provide a unique draw to the field of psychiatry. Although many residency applicants vocalize a desire for psychotherapy training, only 8 of 142 allopathic medical schools in 2020 offered a specific psychotherapy course for fourth-year medical students (Cenoz-Donati et al. 2020). To capitalize on this untapped potential, medical schools should design electives to train fourth-year students in motivational interviewing, cognitive-behavioral therapy, and psychodynamic psychiatry. Residency programs could consider inviting medical students to participate in psychotherapy-focused residency didactics.

Senior electives are a prime opportunity—only partially realized—to introduce students to subspecialties within the field. Among psychiatry fellowships, child psychiatry has the highest percentage of filled positions. It may not be a coincidence that senior electives in child psychiatry are also extremely prevalent, second only to inpatient psychiatry electives (Cenoz-Donati et al. 2020). Introducing more fourth-year electives in other psychiatric subspecialties, such as addiction medicine, brain injury medicine, consult-liaison psychiatry, forensic psychiatry, geriatric psychiatry, hospice and palliative medicine, and sleep medicine, might inspire more future psychiatrists to pursue these fellowships.

The potential of senior electives to benefit students, medical schools, and the field at large should not be underestimated. A medical school's investment in a robust assortment of senior electives continues to pay dividends long after the fourth year of medical school concludes. Strong senior electives may incline students to remain at their home program for residency and may also help to retain visiting medical students. Perhaps most importantly, as students embark on specialty-specific training, they forge skills in fourth-year electives that they will wield throughout residency and will spend a lifetime refining.

Extracurricular Activities and Mentorship

Throughout medical school, extracurricular activities ignite and enhance student interest in psychiatry. Led by medical students with the guidance of a faculty liaison, student interest groups are a landing place for students of all years who are even remotely interested in psychiatry (Seow et al. 2018). Cultivating curiosity, authenticity, and camaraderie among participants, interest groups allow students to evaluate early and discern in time whether psychiatry is the right fit. Interest groups commonly offer a series of lectures that are helpful for enriching the preclerkship neuroscience and behavior curriculum. Additionally, student interest groups provide rich opportunities that may pave the way for a future career in psychiatry: research projects, local volunteering, national conferences, and connections with peers, residents, and faculty who share a dedication to psychiatry. Student interest groups also provide a framework for structured mentorship programs to exist.

Mentorship can play a pivotal role in the formative period of an aspiring psychiatrist. Although medical students highly value mentorship, only about a third of students report having a mentor (Farkas et al. 2019). The authenticity and candor of a mentoring relationship may offer students a welcome respite from the performative aspects of medical school. Effective mentors are readily available and are focused on the mentee: encouraging introspection, tracking progress, identifying strengths, and offering feedback. A mentor's words of encouragement and wisdom may provide an antidote to the imposter syndrome afflicting medical students. Medical schools may consider equipping faculty with formal training in effective mentorship as well as creating intentional mentorship opportunities for underrepresented students in psychiatry. Additionally, students may gain valuable perspective by witnessing how a mentor harmonizes work and life.

Psychiatry not only values the humanity of the patient but also the humanity of the physician. Joining the ranks among radiology, ophthalmology, anesthesiology, and dermatology, psychiatry is now widely considered a "lifestyle" specialty, marked by a favorable integration of life and work, often with relatively light or more favorable hours. Valuing work-life balance is one of the factors most strongly associated with choosing psychiatry (Goldenberg et al. 2017). Students are eager to hear about life outside work. Their specialty selection may be influenced by residents and faculty members demonstrating a dynamic integration of work and life, such as hosting a social event at a faculty member's home or simply including a family photo at the end of a lecture. Faculty should affirm and encourage the particular hobbies, aspirations, or relationships integral to the personal identity of their medical students.

Residency Application Advising

The final stage in promoting student interest in psychiatry comes during the residency application advising process. Students begin making final decisions on specialty applications either late in the third year or early in the fourth year of the curriculum. This period is both exciting and stressful for students, as they are faced with making many life-altering decisions in a short period of time. The guidance of faculty advisors in navigating this process is of the utmost importance

(Thomas et al. 2021). It is imperative that the psychiatry department has an identified individual or group of individuals equipped to support students planning to apply to psychiatry residency. Insufficient advising can lead to students switching to other specialties, whereas comprehensive support can boost the number of students seeking psychiatry residency and improve recruitment to the program at their home institution.

Early in the application preparation season, students benefit from group meetings specifically for students considering applying for psychiatry residency. The meeting invitation may be sent broadly to the class and should be composed so that students with even a modest interest in the specialty are encouraged to attend. The session should be led by an experienced advisor and should provide perspective on recent trends in the residency match and general advice for fourth-year planning. The advisor should acknowledge that students may still be deciding between specialties and should offer advice on how to come to a final decision. A question-and-answer session with a panel of residents may also be helpful, as residents are well equipped to realistically describe the challenges of the application process and residency training.

In addition to group recruitment activities, individual advising sessions are critical in preparing students to apply to residency. These sessions should include a discussion of the student's experiences and motivations leading to an interest in psychiatry, ensuring that the choice of specialty is congruent with the student's interests, skills, and goals. Advisors should offer assistance with personal statements, recommendation letters, application forms, and interview preparation.

Many students will feel confident in their specialty decision at this point in their training, but others may struggle with choosing between psychiatry and other specialties well into their fourth year. Advisors should thus be accessible to undecided students and comfortable frankly discussing the benefits and challenges of a career in psychiatry. Although a degree of recruitment is appropriate in this situation, the advisor must be conscientious of providing unbiased guidance to help students determine which specialty is best for them and their future.

Conclusions

A student's path to psychiatry begins years before medical school and traverses through the preclinical curriculum and clerkships before leading onward to residency. From start to finish, residents, clinical attendings, and teaching faculty are entrusted with playing many different roles throughout this journey. Among an ever-widening stream of qualified applicants, those with aptitude and interest in our specialty should be identified and accepted to medical school. These students may stand out among their peers for their varied academic interests and life experiences complementing their commitment to science. Medical schools should ensure that the preclinical neuroscience and behavior curriculum lays the groundwork for what lies ahead. Most importantly, medical schools should develop and continually improve the psychiatry clerkship, which presents a crucial crossroads for many students. These overarching goals should be paired with a robust commitment to the everyday experience of the student: facilitating extracurricular activities, cultivating mentoring relationships, and advising students as they navigate critical junctures. These collective factors shape a student's choice to advance from general medical training along the specific pathway marked "Psychiatry."

Those embarking on this journey are stepping into the field at an exciting time. As stigma surrounding mental illness continues to dissipate and the demand for psychiatric care rises, the way a medical school fosters a student's interest in psychiatry has never been more important. When successful, these efforts will reflect the very characteristics of our specialty—vibrant and multifaceted both inside and outside the formal educational setting—and will equip our field to provide for the growing needs of the future.

Key Points

- Numerous academic factors influence student interest in various specialties, making it essential for medical schools to create positive experiences for students interested in psychiatry.
- Students' specialty interests evolve during medical training, and interest in psychiatry tends to grow with increased exposure to the specialty.
- Psychiatry has seen a resurgence in popularity among students due to shifting generational priorities and evolving attitudes toward mental health care. However, faculty must continue efforts to sustain this interest in the future.
- The preclinical curriculum is a significant opportunity to shape student perceptions of psychiatry. Faculty should ensure that

psychiatry content is well represented, emphasizing clinical relevance and integration with other medical subjects.
- The clerkship is crucial for sparking student interest in psychiatry. Quality clerkship experiences with diverse clinical exposure, interaction with residents, and engaging didactics positively influence student perceptions of psychiatry.
- Extracurricular activities such as interest groups and mentorship programs play a vital role in nurturing curiosity about psychiatry among students.
- Students interested in psychiatry benefit from specialized group meetings and individual advising sessions. These sessions provide insights into the field, help with application materials, and support those still undecided about their career path.

References

Cenoz-Donati AB, McKinley JC, Schillerstrom JE: A survey of psychiatry course offerings for fourth-year medical students. Acad Psychiatry 44(6):741–744, 2020 32875476

Crowley G, Banerjee S, Page L, Daley S: Factors associated with interest in psychiatry in UK medical students: qualitative study. BJPsych Bull 47(1):48–55, 2023 36731519

Farkas AH, Allenbaugh J, Bonifacino E, et al: Mentorship of US medical students: a systematic review. J Gen Intern Med 34(11):2602–2609, 2019 31485967

Goldenberg MN, Williams DK, Spollen JJ: Stability of and factors related to medical student specialty choice of psychiatry. Am J Psychiatry 174(9):859–866, 2017 28618855

Holt C, Mirvis R, Bao J, et al: Three-year longitudinal follow-up of the psychiatry early experience program (PEEP): gaining and sustaining positive attitudes towards psychiatry in students at a UK medical school. Acad Psychiatry 43(6):600–604, 2019 31372963

Kim J, Blum B, Kaushal S, et al: Impact of psychiatry clerkship rotation in attitudes towards mental illness and psychiatry as a career among medical students. HCA Healthc J Med 4(6):415–420, 2023 38223472

Kumar V: Why a career in psychiatry? Australas Psychiatry 22(3):296–298, 2014 24737266

Lyons Z: Impact of the psychiatry clerkship on medical student attitudes towards psychiatry and to psychiatry as a career. Acad Psychiatry 38(1):35–42, 2014 24464416

National Resident Matching Program: Results and Data: 2023 Main Residency Match. Washington, DC, National Resident Matching Program, 2023.

Available at: https://www.nrmp.org/wp-content/uploads/2023/05/2023-Main-Match-Results-and-Data-Book-FINAL.pdf. Accessed July 21, 2025.

Querido SJ, Vergouw D, Wigersma L, et al: Dynamics of career choice among students in undergraduate medical courses. A BEME systematic review: BEME Guide No. 33. Med Teach 38(1):18–29, 2016 26372112

Russo RA, Dallaghan GB, Balon R, et al: Millennials in psychiatry: exploring career choice factors in generation Y psychiatry interns. Acad Psychiatry 44(6):727–733, 2020 32661946

Russo RA, Griffeth BT, Combs H, et al: Elements of an excellent psychiatry clerkship experience: a survey study of graduating medical students. Acad Psychiatry 45(2):174–179, 2021 33409938

Seow LSE, Chua BY, Mahendran R, Verma S, et al: Psychiatry as a career choice among medical students: a cross-sectional study examining school-related and non-school factors. BMJ Open 8(8):e022201, 2018

Spollen JJ, Beck Dallaghan GL, Briscoe GW, et al: Medical school factors associated with higher rates of recruitment into psychiatry. Acad Psychiatry 41:233–238, 2017

Thomas LA, Schatte D, Briscoe GW, et al: What should faculty advisors know before advising students applying to psychiatry residency. Acad Psychiatry 45(4):506–510, 2021 33765294

Wilbanks L, Spollen JJ, Messias, E: Factors influencing medical school graduates towards a career in psychiatry: analysis from 2011-2013 Association of American Medical Colleges graduation questionnaire. Acad Psychiatry 40:255–260, 2017

Part II

Practical Aspects of Undergraduate Psychiatric Education

5

Theories of Learning and Their Implications for Psychiatric Education

Enoch Ng, M.D., Ph.D.
Hermioni L. Amonoo, M.D., M.P.P., M.P.H.
Shaheen A. Darani, M.D.
Robert Boland, M.D.

Learning in academic medicine is a lifelong endeavor, and how an individual learns may evolve (Panda and Desbiens 2010; Teunissen and Dornan 2008). The factors that promote and foster learning in medicine are intricate. Efforts to comprehend how learning unfolds throughout the medical education journey have delineated intrinsic and extrinsic factors influencing how individuals collect, process, assimilate, and store information to facilitate learning (Boland and Amonoo 2021).

A learning style is a concept wherein individuals possess intrinsic preferences for effective learning based on the mode of instruction or study (Pashler et al. 2008). Learning styles include neurocognitive, personality-based, and metacognitive processes (Boland and Amonoo

2021). The evidence regarding how learning styles are interrelated is mixed, and further work is needed to unpack the impact of learning styles and the factors that contribute to learning across the lifespan of academic medicine learners (Boland and Amonoo 2021; Cuevas 2015; Dekker et al. 2012; Howard-Jones 2014). In this chapter, we review the current evidence in psychology and medical education to assess the hypothesis that customizing instruction methods to an individual's preferred learning styles improves learning outcomes. Finally, we consider how to apply evidence-informed educational principles from cognitive psychology to learners in psychiatry.

Models of Learning Styles

The Meshing Hypothesis

The *visual, auditory, and kinesthetic* (VAK) model is the most studied modality-specific model of learning styles in medicine and across various scientific disciplines (Pashler et al. 2008). The model is occasionally referred to as "VARK," with reading added (Boland and Amonoo 2021). The VARK model hinges on neurocognitive processes and the theory of multiple intelligences, characterized by the ability to problem solve or create according to cultural preferences and values (Gardner 1987). VARK learning styles are assessed through a self-report questionnaire that describes a person's study habits and preferences (Coffield 2004; Dunn and Dunn 1972). Although it has been researched and highly debated for decades (Patil and Newton 2023), the widespread use of VARK learning styles has inspired teachers to tailor their lessons to the preferred learning styles of their learners. Most teachers of academic medicine, however, do not routinely make a formal assessment of medical learners in preparation for lessons, whether in didactic settings such as lectures, bedside teaching during rounds, or with direct patient contact (Lapp et al. 1999; Moreno and Mayer 1999).

VARK can be seen as an instance of the *meshing hypothesis*: it implies that teaching or instructional methods should mesh with a learner's preferred learning style (Rogowsky et al. 2020). Because the brain processes information in a cross-modal fashion based on the interconnectivity of various brain areas (Dekker et al. 2012), the notion of effective teaching based on the meshing hypothesis is a "neuromyth" and not supported by the current understanding of brain functioning (Arbuthnott and Krätzig 2015). The meshing hypothesis has also been scrutinized for underplaying the importance of ability, effort, and content in effective learning (De Fraja et al. 2010; Hallahan 2020). Hence, it is crucial for psychiatric educators to know their learners comprehensively to develop real-time assessments of their teaching. Effective teaching methods may differ for undergraduate and graduate medical education learners (Norman and Lotrecchiano 2021). Indeed, learners across the lifespan of medical education may benefit from a teaching style that uses diverse modalities based on content and context (Lapp et al. 1999).

The Experiential Learning Model

Developed by educational theorist David Kolb, the *experiential learning* model delineates different learning styles in four distinct stages (Fewster-Thuente and Batteson 2018): 1) concrete experience, in which individuals encounter new experiences or revisit situations with a fresh perspective; 2) reflective observation, in which learners reflect on their experiences, focusing on prior assumptions or discrepancies; 3) abstract conceptualization, in which new ideas are formed or existing knowledge is adapted; and 4) active experimentation, in which learners apply and integrate new knowledge into their current environments. Although this model suggests that learners must go through all four stages, the order may vary. For example, a learner with a diverging approach may first experience the situation and then reflect on it before generating new knowledge. A learner with a converging approach may think about an abstract idea before taking action to acquire knowledge. The Kolb model also posits that personality traits influence where a person engages with the stages of learning for acquiring and mastering new knowledge. Additionally, prior work suggests that Kolb's model undergirds teaching interprofessional competencies for health care learners (Fewster-Thuente and Batteson 2018; Murdoch et al. 2017).

The Tripartite Model

Developed by Noel Entwistle, the *tripartite* model emphasizes that motivations significantly impact a preferred learning approach (Entwistle and Ramsden 2015). The learning approaches proposed by this model encompass *deep learning,* in which intrinsic motivation and personal interest drive the learning process. Deep learners are thorough and focus on acquiring comprehensive knowledge. Second, *strategic learning* entails learning motivated by the drive to be successful or have external recognition, such as a good score on a test. Strategic learners tend to prioritize materials and concepts likely to be examined and rewarded, as opposed to seeking comprehensive understanding as in deep learning. Third, *surface learning* occurs when the fear of failure is the primary motivation for learning. These learning styles are not innate but rather preferences for approaches to learning that are sometimes influenced by values, cultural norms, and circumstances surrounding the learning process (Entwistle and Ramsden 2015).

Reviews of Learning Styles in Psychology

Pashler et al. (2008) published an article commissioned by Psychological Science in the Public Interest to assess the evidence for learning styles and their application in school contexts. They started by defining the learning-styles hypothesis (people learn better if taught in a manner that accounts for their learning style), then they outlined four criteria needed to provide evidence supporting the hypothesis (Pashler et al. 2008). First, the study must measure people's learning styles and divide them into groups (e.g., visual versus auditory learners). Second, learners in each group need to be randomly assigned to be taught using different learning methods (e.g., visual versus auditory presentation about the diagnosis of major depressive disorder). Third, after the session, learners across groups must be given the same assessment of their learning. Finally, assessment scores must show a crossover interaction between learning style and instructional method. In other words, the instructional method that leads to optimal assessment scores differs based on learning-style group.

Pashler et al.'s search of the vast psychology literature found only four studies with methods in line with the four criteria needed to test the learning styles hypothesis. Of these, only one marginally supported the hypothesis; three provided no support for the learning styles hypothesis. Pashler et al. (2008) noted that the one study that reported a style-by-treatment interaction had methodological issues that decreased its validity (including using highly derived measures and excluding outliers for unspecified reasons).

More recently, Aslaksen and Lorås (2018) conducted an updated review searching for studies meeting the methodological criteria put forth by Pashler et al. (2008). They searched the literature up to January 2018 and, after scanning 1,215 records, found 10 studies meeting the criteria. In their mini-review, they computed effect sizes pooled across the studies to see whether evidence supports the meshing hypothesis. After pooling 11 experiments from the 10 studies, they found small and nonsignificant effect sizes (g), whether for visual matching ($g = -0.09$) or auditory matching ($g = -0.27$) (note that in psychology and education, practical relevance is defined as $g > 0.4$) (Aslaksen and Lorås 2018). Further, the only study that fully met Pashler's rigorous four criteria was Rogowsky et al. (2015), in which adult learners were first tested on their auditory and visual learning styles and then randomly assigned to be taught the same content using one of two instructional modes, with the same comprehension tests immediately after instruction and 2 weeks later to test for retention. Scores from the comprehension tests demonstrated no interaction between learning style and instructional method, either immediately or at 2 weeks. Hence, Rogowsky et al. (2015) tested the meshing hypothesis in adults and did not find evidence for its validity. In 2020, the authors repeated the same study design and found the same negative results in fifth graders (Rogowsky et al. 2020).

Overall, there is scant empirical literature in psychology to support the idea that teachers should account for individual learning styles to improve learning outcomes. People express and can be tested to have preferences regarding learning, but there is no clear evidence that optimal instruction must account for or even match their preferences. In fact, the studies with the most methodological rigor conducted to date that tested learning styles and the meshing hypothesis have not been supportive of the hypotheses (Aslaksen and Lorås 2018; Pashler et al. 2008; Rogowsky et al. 2015).

Reviews of Learning Styles Literature in Medical Education

Feeley and Biggerstaff (2015) conducted an updated review of the literature on learning styles in light of the increasing diversity among medical students in the United Kingdom. Their review looked at learning *styles* (students' preferred mode of receiving information) and learning *approaches* (the motivations that facilitate learning). In their review of 57 papers, Feeley and Biggerstaff confirmed that learning styles do not appear to affect performance when it comes to exam success. However, students with learning approaches that involve strategic learning (motivated to succeed) and deep learning (intrinsically motivated to learn the material) achieve greater exam success. Their review confirmed that these findings in the literature were not affected by increasing medical student diversity.

Cook et al. (2006) reviewed the literature on cognitive and learning styles (CLSs) in computer-assisted instruction (CAI), particularly how CLSs could inform teaching. Later, Cook (2012) questioned the hypothesis in the prior systematic review that "adaptation to learners' [CLSs] could improve the efficiency of [CAI]." He asserted that CLSs do not substantively affect CAI. To inform his analysis, he used the framework of *aptitude–treatment interactions,* which occur "when a student with attribute 1 (e.g., active learner) learns better with instructional approach A than with approach B, whereas a student with attribute 2 (e.g., reflective learner) learns better with instructional approach B." The aptitude–treatment interactions for teaching imply that "learning will be optimized by using approach A to teach students with attribute 1." In contrast, learning will be optimized by "using approach B to teach students with attribute 2 (i.e., instructional adaptation)" (Cook 2012, p. 778). If all students learn better with one approach, there is no aptitude–treatment interaction, and instructional tailoring is unnecessary. If an aptitude-treatment interaction is present, then tailored instruction affects learning.

In his updated search and reanalysis of the evidence, Cook found that only 9 analyses (14%) of 65 (from 48 studies) demonstrated significant interactions between CLS and the teaching approach (Cook 2012). Hence, if aptitude–treatment interactions with CLSs were present at all, they were rare and insignificant in size. Cook concluded that tailoring teaching to students' CLSs has a limited impact on CAI.

More recently, Newton et al. (2021) reviewed the research on learning styles, principally in health professions education, as an update and extension of their prior 2015 study, which showed that 89% of articles about learning styles were biased in a positive direction. They confirmed that the bias toward learning styles remains high: in 2021, 91% of articles showed a similar positive misrepresentation (Newton et al. 2021)· This neuromyth remained despite the lack of research—and even in health care, where evidence-based practice is highly regarded (Courtney et al. 2019; Sackett et al. 1996).

Davies-Kabir and Aitken (2021) demonstrated the persistence of this neuromyth by using a scoping review to describe how learning styles are represented in the medical education literature. A majority (122 of 176 studies) definitively stated that different students have different learning styles, and 67 studies asserted that instruction should be adapted to students' learning style. Of these definitive statements, only about 50% included citations (Davies-Kabir and Aitken 2021). The authors confirmed Newton et al.'s finding (2021) that positive bias toward learning styles in the medical education literature remains strong despite the lack of evidence for its value; they further showed that its use is regularly touted as an endorsed fact (Davies-Kabir and Aitken 2021).

Thus there is limited empirical evidence in medical education to support that teaching methods should be adapted to students' learning styles to enhance learning. The positive bias in the literature for the value of learning styles is misguided, as it lacks an evidence base, even among health profession educators around the world, where evidence-based principles are fundamental (Newton et al. 2021; Patil and Newton 2023). Learning approaches, however (in contrast to learning styles), may be of value to medical educators: the literature suggests that curricula that support deep and strategic learning may improve learning outcomes (Boland and Amonoo 2021).

More Evidence-Informed Approaches to Teaching

Although there is little evidence for the learning styles hypothesis in the broader psychology or the medical education literature, certain approaches to teaching and learning have received sustained empirical support and are worth considering in designing educational content (Artino et al. 2023).

Funded by the Association for Psychological Science Fund for Teaching and Public Understanding of Psychological Science, Weinstein et al. (2018) compiled six strategies for effective learning supported by decades of evidence in cognitive psychology. The six principles include 1) *spaced practice* (space out studying over time), 2) *retrieval practice* (practice bringing information to mind), 3) *elaboration* (explain and describe with many details), 4) *interleaving* (switch between ideas while studying), 5) use of *concrete examples*, and 6) *dual coding* (combining words and visuals). Winn et al. (2019) applied similar principles (or cognitive learning strategies) in a workshop for pediatric medical educators. In the context of undergraduate psychiatric education, spaced practice and retrieval practice could involve having repeated lower-stakes assessments spread over time to encourage more opportunities for review and recall than one high-stakes final assessment. In building educational content, educators can deliberately interleave contrasting concepts, such as major depressive disorder versus bipolar disorder, elaborating with specific case examples using words and visuals.

Norman and Lotrecchiano (2021) from the Clinical and Translational Science Institutes wrote an excellent primer on translating the learning sciences into principles for the clinical teaching and learning environment. They distilled 11 principles that fit into three categories: 1) acquisition and integration of knowledge (four principles; see next paragraph); 2) social and emotional components of learning (four principles), and 3) elements of skill building (three principles).

The four principles dealing with acquisition and integration of knowledge are prior knowledge, organizing knowledge, cognitive load, and metacognition. To illustrate Norman and Lotrecchiano's principles, we can apply them to teaching psychiatry. When preparing to teach bipolar disorder, psychiatric educators can assess *prior knowledge* and knowledge gaps to best address potential faulty assumptions about the disorder and how it is treated. In addition to teaching the nuances of diagnostic criteria and treatment modalities, educators can scaffold learning by intentionally *organizing knowledge* into helpful schemas such as different bipolar states (e.g., depression, dysthymia, euthymia, hypomania, mania), phases of treatment (e.g., acute treatment phase, maintenance), and categories of medication (e.g., antipsychotics, anticonvulsants). The educator can increase germane *cognitive load* by asking learners to elaborate on and contrast how they might treat a patient differently when they suspect bipolar versus unipolar depression, as well as decrease extraneous cognitive load by providing clear directions and slides or handouts. Educators can harness *metacognition* by providing activities at the middle and end of the instructional period that evaluate students' level of understanding and how it has changed and encourage reflection on areas about which they have further questions (e.g., how to treat anxiety in the context of bipolar disorder).

The social and emotional components of learning are enhanced by attending to motivation, developmental stage, presence, and climate. Educators can improve *motivation* by aligning the curriculum so that tasks are of immediate practical relevance—for example, understanding the risk factors for bipolar disorder while learning how to screen for mood disorders. Accounting for the *developmental stage* of undergraduate learners (relative novices to the area of managing bipolar disorders), it may make sense for educators to provide basic knowledge on its diagnosis and management to scaffold them for later case-based (Thistlethwaite et al. 2012) or problem-based (Dolmans et al.

2005) learning. To foster learners' autonomy, a sense of growing mastery, and a sense of social *presence* among the community of learners, classes should include opportunities to collaborate in small groups and delve further into the nuances of managing bipolar disorder (cued by case vignettes). To promote an inclusive *climate,* the educator can use Universal Design for Learning principles (Rose and Meyer 2002) to choose materials representing diverse experiences and avoid stereotypes.

Psychiatric educators can help learners build skills by attending to the principles of mastery, practice, and feedback. While designing the curriculum, it is important to realize the potential of expert blind spots (Norman and Lotrecchiano 2021) and aspects of diagnosis and treatment that are implicitly known (quickly and intuitively). As such, it may be helpful to collaborate with junior colleagues to clarify the component steps and considerations when choosing specific examples. Making explicit the implicit and breaking down complex skills into components can help learners build *mastery.* Multiple opportunities to *practice* applying skills and knowledge—whether in tests, case-based discussions, role-plays with peers in interview seminars, or simulations with standardized patients—can further build students' skillset. As they practice, giving timely *feedback* with specific action items (such as asking them to review specific sections of clinical practice guidelines) can further optimize learning.

Conclusions

Medical educators in psychiatry strive to cultivate lifelong learning in assessment and treatment by depending on principles of evidence-based medicine (Courtney et al. 2019; Sackett et al. 1996). Aspects of cognitive psychology and neuroscience—how humans best learn information and master skills—should inform how we educate psychiatric learners across the lifespan. Although the belief in learning styles is prevalent within general educational and medical education circles, there is little evidence over decades of research to support modifying instruction to match preferred learning styles (e.g., visual vs. auditory) (Aslaksen and Lorås 2018; Pashler et al. 2008). In contrast, there may be value in promoting learning approaches that facilitate deep learning (Feeley and Biggerstaff 2015). Medical educators best serve learners by applying principles of learning from cognitive psychology with decades of empirical research (Norman and Lotrecchiano 2021; Weinstein et al. 2018; Winn et al. 2019). These evidence-informed educational principles include spaced retrieval practice, elaboration, interleaving, use of concrete examples, dual coding, and attending to the socioemotional elements of learning, skill-building, and mastery.

Key Points

- The concept of *learning styles* proposes that individuals possess intrinsic preferences for effective learning based on the mode of instruction or study.
- There is little evidence supporting the learning styles hypothesis in psychology and in the medical education literature.
- Certain other approaches to teaching and learning have received sustained empirical support and are worth considering in designing educational content.

References

Arbuthnott KD, Krätzig GP: Effective teaching: sensory learning styles versus general memory processes. Compr Psychol 4:06.IT.4.2, 2015

Artino AR Jr, Zafar Iqbal M, Crandall SJ: Debunking the learning-styles hypothesis in medical education. Acad Med 98(2):289, 2023 35544329

Aslaksen K, Lorås H: The modality-specific learning style hypothesis: a mini-review. Front Psychol 9:1538, 2018 30186209

Boland RJ, Amonoo HL: Types of learners. Psychiatr Clin North Am 44(2):141–148, 2021 34049638

Coffield F: Learning Styles and Pedagogy in Post-16 Learning: A Systematic and Critical Review. London, Learning and Skills Research Centre, 2004

Cook DA: Revisiting cognitive and learning styles in computer-assisted instruction: not so useful after all. Acad Med 87(6):778–784, 2012 22534603

Cook DA, Thompson WG, Thomas KG, et al: Impact of self-assessment questions and learning styles in Web-based learning: a randomized, controlled, crossover trial. Acad Med 81(3):231–238, 2006 16501263

Courtney DB, Bennett K, Szatmari P: The forest and the trees: evidence-based medicine in the age of information. J Am Acad Child Adolesc Psychiatry 58(1):8–15, 2019 30577942

Cuevas J: Is learning styles-based instruction effective? A comprehensive analysis of recent research on learning styles. Theory Res Educ 13:308–333, 2015

Davies-Kabir M, Aitken G: Learning styles in medical education: a scoping review [version 1]. MedEdPublish 10:169, 2021

De Fraja G, Oliveira T, Zanchi L: Must try harder: evaluating the role of effort in educational attainment. Rev Econ Stat 92:577–597, 2010

Dekker S, Lee NC, Howard-Jones P, Jolles J: Neuromyths in education: prevalence and predictors of misconceptions among teachers. Front Psychol 3:429, 2012 23087664

Dolmans DHJM, De Grave W, Wolfhagen IHAP, van der Vleuten CPM: Problem-based learning: future challenges for educational practice and research. Med Educ 39(7):732–741, 2005 15960794

Dunn RS, Dunn KJ: Practical Approaches to Individualizing Instruction: Contracts and Other Effective Teaching Strategies. West Nyack, NY, Parker Publishing, 1972

Entwistle N, Ramsden P: Understanding Student Learning (Routledge Revivals). London, Routledge, 1983; reprinted 2015

Feeley A-M, Biggerstaff DL: Exam success at undergraduate and graduate-entry medical schools: is learning style or learning approach more important? A critical review exploring links between academic success, learning styles, and learning approaches among school-leaver entry ("traditional") and graduate-entry ("nontraditional") medical students. Teach Learn Med 27(3):237–244, 2015 26158325

Fewster-Thuente L, Batteson TJ: Kolb's experiential learning theory as a theoretical underpinning for interprofessional education. J Allied Health 47(1):3–8, 2018 29504014

Gardner H: The theory of multiple intelligences. Ann Dyslexia 37(1):19–35, 1987 24234985

Hallahan M: Learning Styles / Fixed vs. Growth Mindset, in The Wiley Encyclopedia of Personality and Individual Differences, 1st Edition. Edited by Carducci BJ, Nave CS, Nave CS. New York, Wiley, 2020, pp 545–549

Howard-Jones PA: Neuroscience and education: myths and messages. Nat Rev Neurosci 15(12):817–824, 2014 25315391

Lapp D, Flood J, Fisher D: Intermediality: how the use of multiple media enhances learning. Read Teach 52:776–780, 1999

Moreno R, Mayer RE: Cognitive principles of multimedia learning: the role of modality and contiguity. J Educ Psychol 91:358–368, 1999

Murdoch NL, Epp S, Vinek J: Teaching and learning activities to educate nursing students for interprofessional collaboration: a scoping review. J Interprof Care 31(6):744–753, 2017 28922039

Newton PM, Najabat-Lattif HF, Santiago G, Salvi A: The learning styles neuromyth is still thriving in medical education. Front Hum Neurosci 15:708540, 2021 34456698

Norman MK, Lotrecchiano GR: Translating the learning sciences into practice: a primer for clinical and translational educators. J Clin Transl Sci 5(1):e173, 2021 34733549

Panda M, Desbiens NA: An "education for life" requirement to promote lifelong learning in an internal medicine residency program. J Grad Med Educ 2(4):562–565, 2010 22132278

Pashler H, McDaniel M, Rohrer D, Bjork R: Learning styles: concepts and evidence. Psychol Sci Public Interest 9(3):105–119, 2008 26162104

Patil A, Newton PM: What happens to the principles of evidence-based practice when clinicians become educators? A case study of the learning styles neuromyth. Med Sci Educ 33(5):1117–1126, 2023 37886285

Rogowsky BA, Calhoun BM, Tallal P: Matching learning style to instructional method: effects on comprehension. J Educ Psychol 107:64–78, 2015

Rogowsky BA, Calhoun BM, Tallal P: Providing instruction based on students' learning style preferences does not improve learning. Front Psychol 11:164, 2020 32116958

Rose DH, Meyer A: Teaching every student in the Digital Age: universal design for learning. Alexandria, VA, Association for Supervision and Curriculum Development, 2002

Sackett DL, Rosenberg WMC, Gray JAM, et al: Evidence based medicine: what it is and what it isn't. BMJ 312(7023):71–72, 1996 8555924

Teunissen PW, Dornan T: Lifelong learning at work. BMJ 336(7645):667–669, 2008 18356236

Thistlethwaite JE, Davies D, Ekeocha S, et al: The effectiveness of case-based learning in health professional education: a BEME systematic review: BEME Guide No. 23. Med Teach 34(6):e421–e444, 2012 22578051

Weinstein Y, Madan CR, Sumeracki MA: Teaching the science of learning. Cogn Res Princ Implic 3(1):2, 2018 29399621

Winn AS, DelSignore L, Marcus C, et al: Applying cognitive learning strategies to enhance learning and retention in clinical teaching settings. MedEdPORTAL 15:10850, 2019 31921996

6

The Psychiatry Clerkship

Jeffrey J. Rakofsky, M.D.
Pochu Ho, M.D.
Jin Y. Han, M.D.

Until the early 20th century, medical education in the United States was neither regulated nor standardized, and clinical clerkships did not exist. Once the first university-based medical school in the United States was established in 1776, one could become a doctor after completing an apprenticeship or a proprietary school (Custers and Cate 2018). The typical length of medical training in the early 19th century was 16 weeks, and medical schools had the power to grant licensure to practice.

In 1847, the American Medical Association (AMA) was founded to "elevate the standard of medical education," including the resolution to separate the licensure bodies from the teaching institutions. AMA created the Council on Medical Education (CME) in 1904 to set standards in medical education (Eaglen 2017). From its first conference, CME established the requirements for entrance into a medical school and standardized medical education to include 2 years of laboratory sciences followed by 2 years of clinical education in a hospital. These recommendations were not uniformly adopted, however; a number of medical schools continued to proliferate without regulation. In response, in 1908, CME commissioned the Carnegie Foundation for the Advancement of Teaching to review medical schools (Beck 2004). The foundation chose Abraham Flexner to lead the survey. After he personally visited and evaluated 147 U.S. and 8 Canadian medical schools, the Flexner Report was published in 1910. It showed that medical schools varied widely in resources (finances, laboratory facilities, and hospitals) (Moll 1968). As a result of the Flexner Report, proprietary schools began to close down.

AMA and the Association of American Medical Colleges (AAMC) independently conducted medical school inspections until 1942, when the Liaison Committee on Medical Education (LCME) was created (Kassebaum 1992). The urgency to form a unifying body to inspect and accredit medical schools was partly out of fear that the Selective Service Act, which advocated for an accelerated medical education to meet the needs of the returning service members from World War II, would threaten the quality of medical schools (Eaglen 2017). Today, the LCME accredits all U.S. and Canadian allopathic medical schools, making full site visits every 8 years that include interviews with the schools' clerkship directors (Association of American Medical Colleges 2025).

One of the Flexner Report's key recommendations was to incorporate hospital teaching into medical school. At the time the report was published, most clinical teaching took the form of ward classes (in which patients were brought to the teaching amphitheater) or section teaching (in which a group of students was brought to the bedside) with a physician. William Osler introduced the concept of clerkship at Johns Hopkins University in 1896. Much like today's clerkship, fourth-year students at Johns Hopkins had direct patient contact on the ward under the direct supervision of residents and attending physicians for 2 months. The students spent the mornings on the wards, attending bedside teaching rounds for 2 hours, and then spent the afternoon in outpatient clinics and lectures. In 1914, the AMA CME recommended that clerkships be the standard of clinical teaching in medical schools (Huddle and Ende 1994).

The first clerkships were in medicine and surgery. The incorporation of psychiatry into medical education was a culmination of events: the closure of asylums, the recognition of the need for psychological care after World War II, the affiliation of medical schools with psychiatric hospitals, the creation of community mental health centers, and the increase in governmental support in research and treatment of mental disorders. The number of medical school graduates entering the field of psychiatry increased exponentially after World War II. From 1945 to 1969, 6.4%–10% of medical graduates entered the field. In the 1970s, however, the number of U.S. graduates going into psychiatry declined (Abraham 2018; Sierles and Taylor 1995). Many factors led to this decline, including a growing student dissatisfaction with the psychiatry training offered during medical school (Light 1975; Nelson 1982). In response to the need for excellence in undergraduate medical education in psychiatry, the Association of Directors of Medical Student Education in Psychiatry (ADMSEP) was formed in 1974 (the first national meeting was held in 1975). The organization's mission includes "supporting, developing, and disseminating research and innovation in teaching methods, content, and evaluation" (Sierles 2007). The work of ADMSEP, in addition to the LCME standards, has helped shape the various elements of the psychiatry clerkship as it exists today.

Clerkship Curriculum

Clerkship Goals and Objectives

The psychiatry clerkship, prepares medical students to diagnose and treat psychiatric illnesses by working directly with patients alongside psychiatric clinicians. The clerkship also exposes students to the field so that they may determine whether this specialty is a good career fit for them.

LCME does not prescribe any specific learning objectives for the psychiatry clerkship; rather, it requires that the learning objectives for each clerkship are known to all medical students, faculty, residents, and others with teaching and assessment responsibilities (Standard 6.1) and that the learning objectives for all clerkships must be linked to the medical school's education program objectives (Standard 8.2) (Association of American Medical Colleges 2023). In 2016, a task force within ADMSEP revised an earlier set of consensus-formed psychiatry learning objectives, resulting in 20 competencies organized into the following 6 categories: medical knowledge, patient care (clinical skills), systems-based practice, interpersonal skills and communication, caring/valuing-professionalism, and practice-based learning (Roman et al. 2016). Within each category is a set of competencies that the student is expected to master, with a developmental framework containing milestones that range from less advanced (preclinical) to more advanced (clinical). These learning objectives are available on the ADMSEP website (https://www.admsep.org/milestones.php).

As stated above, LCME requires that clerkship learning objectives be linked to the medical school's program objectives. These objectives vary from school to school but often integrate the 13 core entrustable professional activities (EPAs) (a series of discrete tasks that trainees are entrusted to perform) with competency domains (categories of observable abilities that integrate knowledge, skills, and attitudes) (Association of American Medical Colleges 2014). The competency domains often include the eight developed as part of the physicians competency resource set: patient care, knowledge for practice, practice-based learning and improvement, interpersonal and communication skills, professionalism, systems-based practice, interprofessional collaboration, and personal and professional development (Englander et al. 2013).

Content

Content for the clerkship should address the learning objectives and can be delivered through bedside teaching, didactics, alternative experiences, and online media. LCME does not provide specific requirements for any individual clerkship but does guide the overall medical school curriculum. It requires the following topics: biomedical, behavioral, and social sciences; organ systems/life cycle/prevention/symptoms/signs/differential diagnosis and treatment planning; scientific method/clinical/translational research; critical judgment/problem-solving skills; societal problems; structural competence, cultural competence, and health inequities; medical ethics; communication skills; and interprofessional collaborative skills. Most of these topics are easily integrated into the psychiatry clerkship curriculum. LCME also requires that the faculty define the types of patients and conditions that students must encounter, the skills to be performed, the settings for those experiences, and the expected levels of responsibility (Association of American Medical Colleges 2023).

ADMSEP developed a list of key diagnoses for medical students, which includes psychiatric conditions that medical students should know following clinical or other intense exposure and addresses this LCME requirement. The key diagnoses include the following: neurodevelopmental disorders; schizophrenia spectrum and other psychotic disorders; bipolar and related disorders; depressive disorders; anxiety disorders; trauma and stressor-related disorders; feeding and eating disorders; somatic symptom and related disorders; substance-related and addictive disorders; neurocognitive disorders; personality disorders; and medication-induced movement disorders and other adverse effects of medications (https://

www.admsep.org/milestones.php?c=keydiagnoses). ADMSEP recommends using this list as a guideline, recognizing that each institution might need to modify the list based on the availability of resources and the patient population it serves.

Much bedside teaching occurs in inpatient units, where students can be integrated into the treatment team and interview patients on their own before or after team rounds. Outpatient settings are sometimes used, but their fast pace often precludes students from interviewing and "taking ownership" of the patient; thus their experience may be best described as "shadowing." Students also receive bedside teaching in consultation/liaison teams, on which they can more richly appreciate the interface of psychiatric illnesses with medical diseases. Partial hospital programs and psychiatric emergency rooms can also be good settings for bedside teaching.

Didactics can occur on one weekday or throughout the week. Didactics serve to standardize the learning experience, compensating for different student placement sites with different patient populations, with or without residents, and with attendings who have expertise in specific areas of psychiatry. The clerkship learning objectives can determine the didactic topics and can be provided by the clerkship director, department faculty, or chief/senior residents. Given the age of medical students, teachers should incorporate adult learning strategies and practical materials, and the lectures should differ from those given during the preclinical years.

Alternative experiences may include a half- or full-day opportunity to observe specialty clinical work, such as electroconvulsive therapy, transcranial magnetic stimulation, ketamine infusions, behavioral health court, or methadone clinics—areas of psychiatry that they are not likely to see at their primary sites. Online media such as learning modules, podcasts, and videos may be additional ways to deliver content included in the learning objectives.

The ADMSEP Clinical Simulation Initiative (CSI) Committee was formed in 2010 to develop free, high-quality, interactive, web-based learning modules to complement clinical experiences. These peer-reviewed modules are available via the ADMSEP website (https://www.admsep.org/csi-emodules.php?c=emodules-description).

Length and Structure

The length of the psychiatry clerkship determines the amount of didactic and clinical experiences students will receive. In 2006, ADMSEP published a position statement that the psychiatry clerkship must be 6 weeks or longer. According to a 2016 ADMSEP membership survey, the mean length of the rotation was 5.12 weeks; 40% percent of the respondents reported a 4-week clerkship; 45% reported having a 6-week clerkship; five programs had a 5-week clerkship; and three programs had a 7-week clerkship (Association of Directors of Medical Student Education in Psychiatry 2006; Thomas et al. 2018). Students may be assigned to a single clinical site (such as an inpatient unit) for the duration of the rotation, or they can be assigned to rotate through multiple sites (e.g., alternating inpatient and ambulatory experiences). The advantage of being at one site for the entire duration is that the clinical team has more time to develop trust in the students and incorporate them in decision-making. Also, orienting the students is less burdensome if the rotation is longer, and the attending has more opportunities to see the student perform and thus provide a more valid assessment. The advantage of the alternating structure, in contrast, is that the student gains more exposure to the varied psychiatric conditions of both settings and opportunities to get feedback and evaluations from more educators.

Some institutions have developed longitudinal integrated clerkships, which provide students with curriculum continuity and longitudinal relationships with patients and faculty. Outcomes for students enrolled in these programs equal or exceed those in a traditional rotation block structure (Poncelet et al. 2011). The 2016 ADMSEP survey reported that although 61% of respondents had a longitudinal integrated clerkship at their institution, only 25% included psychiatry; 13% reported that their psychiatry clerkship was integrated with another individual clerkship. Six of seven respondents indicated separate clerkship directors and coordinators for the two combined clerkships (Thomas et al. 2018).

Assessments, Feedback, and Evaluations

LCME requires medical schools to have a centralized system that uses various measures to assess students' acquisition of skills, knowledge, behaviors, and attitudes included in the program objectives. Several assessment tools have been published and used for this purpose; the LCME requires that one of these assessments be narrative, describing the student's performance and noncognitive achievements (Association of American Medical Colleges 2023). Site attendings may use a score sheet or assessment form to rate a student's clinical performance during the rotation. The items to be scored can include entrustable professional activities, specific skills, or competencies.

The scale for scoring could be norm referenced, criterion referenced, or an entrustment scale, which uses narrative descriptors that reflect real-world judgments about a student's readiness for practice (Rekman et al. 2016). Thus a norm-referenced scale would assess the student compared with, for example, the average third-year medical student at a given institution. A criterion-referenced scale would assess the student according to a given standard (e.g., using a cut score to determine mastery, proficiency, or needing improvement) (Burkett 2018). Other assessments include written exams, such as the National Board of Medical Examiners (NBME) Psychiatry Subject Exam, which measures the student's knowledge and ability to diagnose and treat psychiatric illnesses. Observed structured clinical examinations (OSCEs) are also used in clerkships (Vitiello et al. 2021). They combine standardization of the exam experience for students with direct assessment of clinical skills, such as delivering upsetting news or building rapport with a patient. Other assessments may involve narrative reflections, patient write-ups, or a professionalism score.

LCME requires that faculty provide students with formative feedback early enough during the clerkship (midpoint or earlier) to allow the student time to improve. Final grades must be submitted within 6 weeks of the end of the clerkship (Association of American Medical Colleges 2023). The summative evaluation combines assessment performance to measure overall proficiency in the rotation. Increasingly, medical schools are moving away from traditional letter grades and toward pass/fail or honors/pass/fail grade reporting (faculty members determine appropriate cut scores). The clerkship director must also determine the appropriate weights for each assessment (clinical performance vs. written exam). Grading committees are increasingly used to improve grading fairness, but they have limitations (Frank et al. 2019).

Role of Clerkship Director

The clerkship director must have a varied skillset to run the clerkship effectively. They are nearly always psychiatrists and must stay abreast of the latest developments in the field. They must make hiring and firing decisions for their clerkship team, including the clerkship coordinator and, if a program has them, associate and assistant clerkship directors. They must manage the team effectively, which requires them to ensure accountability, incorporate feedback and ideas from the team, and provide annual feedback. They must design the curriculum, identify the learning objectives, and determine which assessment tools and evaluation framework to use. They must address professionalism issues that arise among students and faculty. They must network and reach out to psychiatrists within and outside the academic institution to create new rotation sites, recruit new lecturers for didactics, and find faculty to help grade exams. Finally, they must ensure comparable educational experiences and equivalent assessment methods across all sites to ensure that all students achieve the same objectives (Association of American Medical Colleges 2023). According to the Alliance for Clinical Education's collaborative statement from its member organizations on expectations for clerkship directors, there should be a minimum of 50% full-time-equivalent (FTE) salary support for clerkship directors (Morgenstern et al. 2021). According to the 2021 ADMSEP membership survey, 28.5% of respondents received 41%–50% salary support; 31% received 20% or less (Russo et al. 2022).

Challenges and Future Directions

Vertical Integration

Several medical schools have implemented strategies to vertically integrate foundational sciences and clinical courses. They identified several barriers, including shortened length of rotations, increased productivity pressure on faculty while managing a busy schedule, and limited faculty development integrating basic and clinical sciences. It is also well known that the knowledge of basic sciences diminishes over time unless there is a deliberate effort to review the material and incorporate the knowledge into routine practice and teaching. During clinical courses, there is an emphasis on teaching and assessing clinical reasoning, but the opportunity to incorporate basic sciences into the formulation is often lacking. According to a multi-institution collaborative article, integrating basic and clinical sciences into clerkships faced several challenges at the program, clerkship, bedside, and assessment levels (Daniel et al. 2021).

Shortened Clerkships

Over the last few years, psychiatry clerkships have been shortened. This trend continues, and there is limited research on the implications of these shortened clerkships for medical students obtaining clinical core competencies in psychiatry. The main concern is the impact on the U.S. health care system, since there is a projected shortage of psychiatrists despite the efforts to expand the specialty workforce (Satiani et al. 2018). Perhaps the shortened duration will attract fewer students to the field. Many future primary care clinicians, hospitalists, and emergency department physicians will face significant challenges because of limited access to psychiatric consultations and referrals. Additionally, if the psychiatric training received by these front-line providers is reduced owing to a shortened clerkship, they will feel less confident providing first-line treatments, creating even more access issues.

Grade Fairness

Despite curricular standards for accreditation, there is no current standardization of clerkship grading systems. This variability results in unique institutional approaches to grading fairness, and despite the efforts of clerkship directors across the nation, student perception of grading fairness remains low (Bullock et al. 2019). Documented approaches to improve clerkship grading fairness include moving to a more competency-based system, deemphasizing the NBME, and using grading committees (Bullock et al. 2022; Schilling 2019).

Conclusions

The psychiatry clerkship is a core clinical course during medical school, and its course objectives must align with the school's main objectives. The clerkship director should develop the course based on recommendations provided by ADMSEP, which provides a set of learning goals and competencies and a list of the most important clinical cases for students to meet course requirements. Rotation length varies, but ADMSEP's official position is that it last at least 6 weeks. The schedule depends on the resources available. Ideally, a combination of inpatient and ambulatory site assignments will facilitate exposure to broader diagnostic categories and clinical experiences. Didactic content should also align with the course objectives and key diagnostic categories as recommended by ADMSEP, but additional topics could be introduced depending on clerkship length. ADMSEP CSI modules are good resources to supplement the learning curve for medical students.

Assessment and evaluation tools should capture the student's clinical knowledge, clinical skills, and professionalism. The NBME

Psychiatry Subject Exam and OSCEs are commonly used in addition to clinical evaluations. Some institutions also include write-ups and professionalism scoring. The clinical evaluation form captures the student's clinical performance during the rotation. Depending on the grading system, the evaluation scale could be criterion referenced, norm referenced, entrustment style, or a combination. Regular feedback regarding professionalism and clinical skills is a key tool to help students grow during the clerkship and is generally provided verbally or in writing.

The effectiveness of the clerkship director correlates with a well-managed clerkship, which requires coordination of all educational resources while continuously implementing strategies to improve the quality of the curriculum. The job requires sufficient support from the school and the department.

Ongoing research within the field of psychiatry has led to a growing number of treatment options. Advancements in neuroscience, psychology, and pharmacology have played a key role in these discoveries. Therefore, optimally integrating basic sciences into our clerkships is more important than ever as we engage in curriculum reform.

Key Points

- Psychiatry clerkship objectives must align with the medical school's core educational program objectives.
- ADMSEP provides guidelines related to psychiatry clerkship learning goals and competencies and a list of key diagnoses for medical students.
- The length of the psychiatry clerkship varies, but ADMSEP recommends at least 6 weeks.
- An inpatient and ambulatory combined rotation provides broader exposure to key diagnostic categories (vs. a single-site rotation).
- The NBME Psychiatry Subject Exam and OSCEs are commonly used in addition to clinical evaluation forms.
- Quality feedback about a student's clinical skills is required and generally given verbally or in writing.
- Grading systems and evaluation scales may be criterion referenced, norm referenced, entrustment style, or a combination.
- Optimal integration of basic sciences into our clerkships is an important milestone for curriculum reform.

References

Abraham TH: Psychiatry in American medical education: the case of Harvard's medical school, 1900–1945. Can Bull Med Hist 35(1):63–93, 2018 29661008

Association of American Medical Colleges: Core Entrustable Professional Activities for Entering Residency, Curriculum Developers' Guide, 2014. Available at: https://store.aamc.org/downloadable/download/sample/sample_id/63/%20. Accessed June 2, 2025.

Association of American Medical Colleges; American Medical Association: LCME Functions and Structure of a Medical School. Standards for Accreditation of Medical Education Programs Leading to the MD Degree. Liaison Committee on Medical Education, 2023. Available at: https://lcme.org/wp-content/uploads/2025/03/2024-25-Functions-and-Structure_2025-03-07.docx. Accessed June 2, 2025.

Association of American Medical Colleges; American Medical Association: LCME Rules of Procedure. Liaison Committee on Medical Education, 2025. Available at: https://lcme.org/wp-content/uploads/2025/03/Rules-of-Procedure_2025-03-07.docx. Accessed June 2, 2025.

Association of Directors of Medical Student Education in Psychiatry; Executive Council of the Associaton of Academic Psychiatry: The psychiatry clerkship: a position statement on the length of the psychiatry clerkship. Acad Psychiatry 30(2):103, 2006 16609113

Beck AH: The Flexner report and the standardization of American medical education. JAMA 291(17):2139–2140, 2004 15126445

Bullock JL, Lai CJ, Lockspeiser T, et al: In pursuit of honors: a multi-institutional study of students' perceptions of clerkship evaluation and grading. Acad Med 94(11S):S48–S56, 2019

Bullock JL, Seligman L, Lai CJ, et al: Moving toward mastery: changes in student perceptions of clerkship assessment with pass/fail grading and enhanced feedback. Teach Learn Med 34(2):198–208, 2022 34014793

Burkett T: Norm-Referenced Testing and Criterion-Referenced Testing, in The TESOL Encyclopedia of English Language Teaching. New York, Wiley and Sons, 2018

Custers EJFM, Cate OT: The history of medical education in Europe and the United States, with respect to time and proficiency. Acad Med 93(3S):S49–S54, 2018

Daniel M, Morrison G, Hauer KE, et al: Strategies from 11 U.S. medical schools for integrating basic science into core clerkships. Acad Med 96(8):1125–1130, 2021 33394668

Eaglen RH: Academic Quality and Public Accountability in Academic Medicine: The 75-Year History of the LCME. Washington, DC, Liaison Committee on Medical Education, 2017. Available at: https://www.lcme.org/wp-content/uploads/filebase/articles/October-2017-The-75-Year-History-of-the-LCME_COLOR.pdf. Accessed June 2, 2025.

Englander R, Cameron T, Ballard AJ, et al: Toward a common taxonomy of competency domains for the health professions and competencies for physicians. Acad Med 88(8):1088–1094, 2013 23807109

Frank AK, O'Sullivan P, Mills LM, et al: Clerkship grading committees: the impact of group decision-making for clerkship grading. J Gen Intern Med 34(5):669–676, 2019 30993615

Huddle TS, Ende J: Osler's clinical clerkship: origins and interpretations. J Hist Med Allied Sci 49(4):483–503, 1994 7844340

Kassebaum DG: Origin of the LCME, the AAMC-AMA partnership for accreditation. Acad Med 67(2):85–87, 1992 1547000

Light D Jr: The impact of medical school on future psychiatrists. Am J Psychiatry 132(6):607–610, 1975 1124803

Moll W: History of American medical education. Br J Med Educ 2(3):173–181, 1968 4879055

Morgenstern BZ, Roman BJB, DeWaay D, et al: Expectations of and for clerkship directors 2.0: a collaborative statement from the Alliance for Clinical Education. Teach Learn Med 33(4):343–354, 2021 34294018

Nelson B: Psychiatry's anxious years: decline in allure as a career leads to self-examination. Bol Asoc Med P R 74(10):304–305, 1982 6963894

Poncelet A, Bokser S, Calton B, et al: Development of a longitudinal integrated clerkship at an academic medical center. Med Educ Online 16, 2011 21475642

Rekman J, Gofton W, Dudek N, et al: Entrustability scales: outlining their usefulness for competency-based clinical assessment. Acad Med 91(2):186–190, 2016 26630609

Roman B, Schatte D, Frank J, et al: The ADMSEP Milestones Project. Acad Psychiatry 40(2):314–316, 2016 25894731

Russo RA, Blazek MC, Thomas LA: The 2021 Survey of the Association of Directors of Medical Student Education in Psychiatry. Acad Psychiatry 46(3):403–404, 2022 34586596

Satiani A, Niedermier J, Satiani B, Svendsen DP: Projected workforce of psychiatrists in the United States: a population analysis. Psychiatr Serv 69(6):710–713, 2018 29540118

Schilling DC: Using the clerkship shelf exam score as a qualification for an overall clerkship grade of honors: a valid practice or unfair to students? Acad Med 94(3):328–332, 2019 30188368

Sierles FS: The Association of Directors of Medical Student Education in Psychiatry. Acad Psychiatry 31(2):107–109, 2007 17344443

Sierles FS, Taylor MA: Decline of U.S. medical student career choice of psychiatry and what to do about it. Am J Psychiatry 152(10):1416–1426, 1995 7573579

Thomas LA, Dallaghan GB, Balon RM: The 2016 Survey of the Association of Directors of Medical Student Education in Psychiatry. Acad Psychiatry 42(3):366–370, 2018 29299832

Vitiello E, Doctor D, Lindner S, et al: A novel approach to standardization and resident involvement in the psychiatry clerkship OSCE. Acad Psychiatry 45(2):190–194, 2021 33420701

7

Psychiatry Electives

Julie Williams, M.S., M.D.
Elijah Li, M.D.

Medical electives are complex, having a diversity of objectives and targeted students. Added to this complexity is the variability of medical school curricula. For example, some schools may not allow for the selection of electives until the student's fourth year; others allow elective enrollment as a first-year student. Although the design of an elective can be a daunting task for any faculty member, the ability to share one's expertise with a passionate medical student is a gift. This chapter explores the complicated process of elective design.

Elective Types

Electives fall into three primary categories: foundational, research, and clinical (Figure 7.1). Many students will have limited clinical exposure before enrollment; foundational electives are usually designed for a first- or second-year medical student who has some curiosity about the field, if not a budding interest. Foundational electives are best designed to have broad applicability to many fields in medicine. Behavioral topics such as wellness, professionalism, and human sexuality, which are often introduced in basic science courses, can be explored in greater detail. Active learning tools such as team-based learning activities or discussion groups increase student engagement.

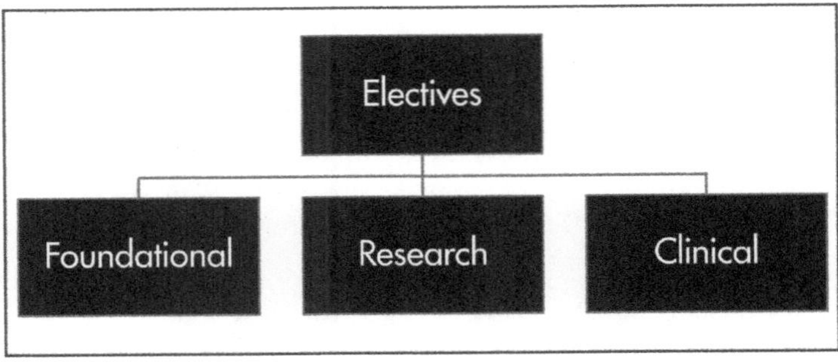

Figure 7.1 Elective types

Research electives can be based in the clinic or the laboratory. As the residency match in psychiatry becomes increasingly competitive, involvement in scholarship activities is one way that applicants can stand out among their peers. Although a student may not be able to complete a research project start to finish within a few weeks during an elective, exposure to the investigative process and initiation of a longer-term project is immensely beneficial.

Clinical electives provide students with unique clinical experiences outside of the core psychiatry clerkship. The goals of electives may change depending on length and timing, but recruitment into psychiatry remains a primary aim. These electives are the primary focus of this chapter.

Goals

The primary goal of any elective is to expand a student's knowledge base in an area of interest, and the unique educational objectives of each course should remain in focus. A major point of emphasis by the Association of Directors of Medical Student Education in Psychiatry (ADMSEP) is establishing appropriate objectives for the psychiatry core clerkship; this should be no different for psychiatry electives (Brodkey et al. 1997). In addition, however, there are other less concrete goals that often accompany elective courses (Figure 7.2).

First, electives serve as a tool to recruit interested students into the field. Specialty choices can be quite unstable in medical school as students explore and gain experience in all fields of medicine. Clinical electives have been shown to have a positive or reaffirming impact on

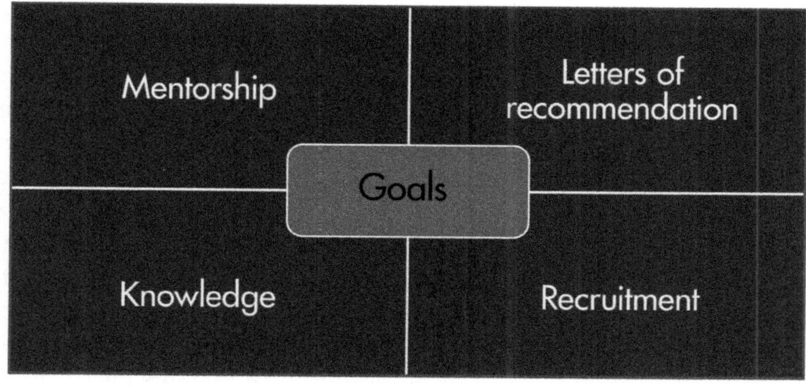

Figure 7.2 Elective Course Goals

a student's ultimate career decision (Mihalynuk et al. 2006). Zimny and Sata (1986) found that clinical electives in psychiatry were the most influential factor during medical school in determining whether a student wound up choosing a career in psychiatry. Similarly, Farooq et al. (2013) found that enrichment activities such as psychiatry electives and psychiatry-focused clubs were the strongest factors associated with choosing psychiatry as a specialty.

Finding mentorship is a top priority for many medical students engaging in elective courses. Students who enroll in research electives early in their medical school careers can develop long-lasting professional relationships with their attending mentors. Wrenn et al. (2016) described a specific academic psychiatry elective in which mentors are assigned to students with the primary goal of fostering academic projects and career advising. Clinically, electives offer students the opportunity to engage in a unique treatment setting to help decide whether the setting is a good fit while also introducing them to practicing physicians who can guide them on their career paths.

Students also engage in electives to gain experience and clinical knowledge. Some electives may provide an experience more in-depth than "bread-and-butter" psychiatry, such as rotating on a traditional inpatient unit, and the student's role is elevated from that of a core clerkship rotation. Whereas a core clerkship is expected to educate students on general psychiatry, including the diagnosis and treatment of a variety of disorders, electives can focus on a particular area of interest. For example, a student may achieve greater exposure to child psychiatry, forensics, addiction psychiatry, or specific treatment settings such as a consult service or emergency center. This knowledge and experience can aid the student in the transition to residency.

Finally, as the residency application cycle approaches, students often search for clinicians who can provide robust letters of recommendation. Currently, residency directors consider letters of recommendation one of the less meaningful components of an application (MacLean et al. 2011). As the psychiatry residency match process grows more competitive, however, strong letters of recommendation are increasingly important for a student's application. ADMSEP recently developed a standardized letter of recommendation in hopes of producing letters that benefit not only the student, but residency program directors as well, in the search for optimum candidates for their program. The hope is that a standardized letter of recommendation will enable programs to sift through the increasing numbers of applicants more quickly (Association of Directors of Medical Student Education in Psychiatry 2023).

Duration

In 2006, ADMSEP published a statement that core clerkships should be at least 6 weeks in length, the rationale being that the skills needed to appropriately evaluate, diagnose, and manage psychiatric disorders are neither easily nor quickly learned (Association of Directors of Medical Student Education in Psychiatry 2006). Furthermore, for students not planning to pursue a career in psychiatry, a junior psychiatry clerkship may be the last opportunity to receive formal training in general care for prevalent psychiatric disorders and to clear up any misperceptions (Brodkey et al. 1997). Although the guidelines for the optimal duration of a clerkship are clear, identifying the ideal duration for electives can be challenging because of their complexity (Cenoz-Donati et al. 2020).

Although electives that are shorter (less than 4 weeks) provide less exposure to a field, they can provide an excellent opportunity to introduce particular concepts at a relatively low commitment for students. Medical students at the University of California San Francisco are required to participate in three 2-week electives during their clerkship year. According to data on the impact of these short electives, students agreed that at least one elective was instrumental in solidifying their specialty choice. Students also felt that the electives were helpful in developing relationships in their field of interest and learning skills important for core clerkships (Sheu et al. 2022). Providing students with the opportunity to take short psychiatry electives before or during their clerkship years can help with recruitment for the field and also helps students perform better during core clerkships, which can be a major factor in successfully obtaining a residency interview (National Resident Matching Program 2022).

The Icahn School of Medicine at Mount Sinai developed a 4-week "integrated clinical neuroscience" curriculum available for students after their neurology and psychiatry core clerkships to gain additional understanding of the integration between the two fields. The course included a series of week-long subspecialty rotations with an underlying goal of attracting students to the two fields. Postrotation surveys, however, showed that students were less likely to choose either specialty after participating in the course (Popeo and Goldstein 2016). Thus, providing multiple short rotations can increase the breadth of exposure, but 1 week is likely too short to influentially impact student specialty selection.

An elective that is too short in duration simply may not provide enough opportunities to successfully address the objectives of the elective; in addition, students are less able to showcase the progression of their skills. This opportunity to demonstrate growth is further reduced if engaging with multiple different faculty members while on rotation (limiting the duration of experience with each attending). Students hoping to gain deeper insights into a particular aspect of psychiatry may not be satisfied with a shorter elective. The Mayo Clinic School of Medicine found that scores on the National Board of Medical Examiners (NBME) shelf exam decreased after the clerkship was shortened from 6 to 3 weeks, suggesting that students were less knowledgeable regarding psychiatric topics (Bostwick and Alexander 2012). Clerkships and electives are different, of course, but giving students enough time on an elective to adequately explore their interests is an important consideration. Electives designed for students already planning to pursue a career in that specialty tend to be longer in duration. Additionally, given that many students hope to receive a strong letter of recommendation, it is important for the electives to be long enough that potential letter writers can satisfactorily assess the student.

Ultimately, when determining the duration for a psychiatry elective, the purpose of the elective and the characteristics of students likely to enroll in the elective must be major points of consideration. Electives that introduce students to the field may be shorter, and it makes sense for students to enroll in these electives early in their medical school education. Electives that are more advanced and primarily designed for students planning to pursue a career in psychiatry likely need to be longer so that learning objectives are sufficiently addressed and students garner the greatest benefit from their enrollment.

Grading

Medical schools across the nation use a variety of grading constructs. Many schools are progressing toward a pass/fail system to emphasize medical student competency and reduce unnecessary angst and competition among peers. Many electives, particularly those designed for medical students in their preclinical years, follow a pass/fail grading system (or honors/high pass/pass). Others, often designed for enrollment after the student's core clerkship, follow a more traditional letter grading system (i.e., A/B/C/F). Letter grading offers potential benefits, such as an opportunity to show improvement in the field of choice if they previously underperformed. It also provides an opportunity for residency applicants to stand out from their peers. Conversely, a graded system may result in students choosing a limited subset of electives that have historically conferred higher-than-average grades as the student attempts to curate a residency application that highlights their performance in the best light.

Away Electives

Hosting students from visiting institutions is an honor that should not be taken lightly. As residency applications become increasingly competitive, students pursuing psychiatry are looking for opportunities to establish relationships with prospective programs and obtain letters of recommendation. In turn, away electives provide an opportunity for programs to highlight the excellent education available in their departments.

One of the largest barriers to hosting students from other institutions is credentialing. For example, many hospital systems require weeks of advance notice, which often is not possible due to rapidly changing enrollments. Applications for away electives are most often submitted through the Visiting Student Learning Opportunities (VSLO) system. Application cycles open twice a year, corresponding to fall and spring academic semesters. Each institution and department determines its own timeline and criteria for acceptance. While this creates advantageous flexibility for the individual departments, it can often result in unnecessary angst for students—for example, the student's home institution may forbid scheduling changes within a certain time limit, but the hosting institution does not make selections until close to the term start date. Another barrier is limited enrollment numbers as institutions navigate meeting the educational needs of varied learners.

Student Cases

In this section, we discuss three hypothetical students and what they may desire from their elective opportunities.

Dan

Dan is a second-year medical student. He had little experience of mental health before medical school, but as he progressed, he enjoyed his behavioral science courses more and more, and he has started to consider a career in psychiatry. As his psychiatry clerkship approaches, he has concerns surrounding his performance, given that many of his classmates seem to have more familiarity with the subject matter. He notes that some of his classmates applied to medical school already knowing they wanted to pursue psychiatry. His medical school allows him to enroll in electives before engaging in his core clerkships as a third-year student.

Depending on his schedule flexibility, as determined by his medical school, Dan can consider enrolling in a preclinical elective versus a research elective. Because of the innate characteristics of the investigative process, research electives tend to engage the student for a longer duration (4 weeks or longer). Meanwhile, with appropriately limited learning objectives, foundational electives may require only 2 weeks. In addition, Dan may consider taking a 2-week clinical elective with the primary goal of receiving an introduction to psychiatry and building interview skills, which will provide an advantage in his core clerkships.

Mirasol

Mirasol is a rising fourth-year medical student. She entered medical school with the explicit goal of becoming a psychiatrist. She performed well on her core clerkship, and she plans to apply to residency in the fall.

Mirasol would benefit from enrolling in longer 4-week clinical electives, preferably in a unique setting of interest. This will help her expand her knowledge base in preparation for residency. It will also allow her to establish a working relationship with a clinical attending physician who could write a robust letter of recommendation for her application.

Ravi

Ravi is a third-year medical student who anticipated pursuing another specialty. After completing his core psychiatry clerkship in the middle of his third year, he decided to pursue psychiatry. He had an average performance in his clerkship for his level of training. He is concerned that by choosing psychiatry just a few short months before residency applications are due, he has put himself at a disadvantage.

Ravi would most benefit from mentorship. He should enroll in 4-week clinical and research electives if his schedule allows. These courses will allow him to interact with multiple key faculty members who could guide him through his career and write him a letter of recommendation when he applies for residency.

Conclusions

Electives are a critical component of medical student education. They play a key role in both student education and recruitment. Although they are complex in design, the flexibility inherent to these courses allows faculty the opportunity to educate students in an environment tailored to their specific goals.

Key Points

- Psychiatric elective design is complex because of the variability in type, duration, goals, and grading schema.
- Clarification of students' needs is key to appropriate design.
- Electives can be helpful to provide education, solidify a budding interest in the field, establish mentorship, and provide opportunities to request letters of recommendation.
- Shorter electives tend to be best for students who are unsure of their selected field of study for residency; longer electives tend to benefit students who have decided to pursue psychiatry as a career.

- A pass/fail grading system establishes competency; a letter-graded system allows for students to demonstrate excellence among peers.
- Away electives provide an opportunity for programs to highlight their unique clinical sites and for students to establish relationships and demonstrate skill outside of their home programs.

References

Association of Directors of Medical Student Education in Psychiatry; Executive Council of the Association of Academic Psychiatry: The psychiatry clerkship: a position statement on the length of the psychiatry clerkship. Acad Psychiatry 30(2):103, 2006 16609113

Association of Directors of Medical Student Education in Psychiatry: The proposal of a standardized letter of recommendation for psychiatry residency applicants. Available at: https://www.admsep.org/subpages/studentmatch/slor-proposed.pdf. Accessed October 21, 2023.

Bostwick JM, Alexander C: Shorter psychiatry clerkship length is associated with lower NBME psychiatry shelf exam performance. Acad Psychiatry 36(3):174–176, 2012 22751816

Brodkey AC, Van Zant K, Sierles FS: Educational objectives for a junior psychiatry clerkship: development and rationale. Acad Psychiatry 21(4):179–204, 1997 24435646

Cenoz-Donati AB, McKinley JC, Schillerstrom JE: A survey of psychiatry course offerings for fourth-year medical students. Acad Psychiatry 44(6):741–744, 2020 32875476

Farooq K, Lydall GJ, Bhugra D: What attracts medical students towards psychiatry? A review of factors before and during medical school. Int Rev Psychiatry 25(4):371–377, 2013 24032490

MacLean LM, Alexander G, Oja-Tebbe N: Letters of recommendation in residency training: what do they really mean? Acad Psychiatry 35(5):342–343, 2011 22106495

Mihalynuk T, Leung G, Fraser J, et al: Free choice and career choice: clerkship electives in medical education. Med Educ 40(11):1065–1071, 2006 17054615

National Resident Matching Program: At-a-glance program director survey. November 28, 2022. Available at: https://www.nrmp.org/match-data/2022/09/results-of-the-2022-nrmp-program-director-survey/. Accessed October 23, 2023.

Popeo DM, Goldstein MA: Design and piloting of an integrated neuroscience elective for medical students in their clinical clerkships. Acad Psychiatry 40(2):359–362, 2016 25749921

Sheu L, Goglin S, Collins S, et al: How do clinical electives during the clerkship year influence career exploration? A qualitative study. Teach Learn Med 34(2):187–197, 2022 33792448

Wrenn G, Johnson V, Edukuye O, Seawell M: Academic psychiatry elective: mentored academic leadership development for medical students. Acad Psychiatry 40(3):434–435, 2016 26590141

Zimny GH, Sata LS: Influence of factors before and during medical school on choice of psychiatry as a specialty. Am J Psychiatry 143(1):77–80, 1986 3942291

8

Psychotherapy Education for Medical Students

Amy S. Brenner, M.S.W., LCSW-S
Adam M. Brenner, M.D.

> "All physicians...are continually practicing psychotherapy, even when you have no intention of doing so and are not aware of it."
> —Sigmund Freud, 1904

Many people would instinctively deem Freud's suggestion as impossible. Not only will many doctors never need to practice psychotherapy (they might argue), but packed training schedules leave no room to teach an entirely new discipline.

Teaching medical students to practice an entire extra specialty might be beyond the time frame available or the competencies necessary, but teaching medical students a set of basic psychotherapeutic skills deserves a careful second look. Mental health affects every patient in every specialty, and instruction in psychotherapeutic skills helps future doctors meet patients where they are. Medical illnesses are themselves affected by social determinants of health, such as adverse childhood experiences or current economic distress. Learning how to effectively support a patient in the face of sociocultural stressors is a valuable skill that can potentially alter the trajectory of a wide array of medical conditions. Understanding how to respond psychotherapeutically—outside the context of formal psychotherapy—can be a great benefit to both clinician and patient.

Literature over the decades does describe efforts to teach medical students psychotherapy. Truong et al. (2015) provided a systematic review of the literature on psychotherapy instruction for medical students and residents. They found only two studies regarding interventions for medical students that met their inclusion criteria, and even those studies had significant methodological problems (Truong et al. 2015). The literature generally consists of uncontrolled trials and anecdotal reports. Nonetheless, some common themes emerge.

What are the potential benefits to teaching basic psychotherapeutic skills to medical students? First, such instruction may help recruit medical students into psychiatry. Second, it may help them understand when patients might need referrals for psychiatric treatment. Third, it may help with the general development of empathy. Fourth, and perhaps most crucial, it can show medical students how to support so-called difficult patients—those who are uncooperative during treatment or whose diagnoses have led to difficult interpersonal patterns.

Recruiting

Psychiatry has increased in popularity in recent years, and rarely do general psychiatry slots go unfilled in "the match" (connecting fourth-year medical students with residency programs). Still, we cannot afford to be complacent about recruiting; we continue to have a significant workforce shortage in the context of growing mental health demands (Satiani et al. 2018). A survey by the Substance Abuse and Mental Health Services Administration (SAMHSA) (2018) found that less than half (46.6%) of adults needing treatment were able to access it.

Many medical students who were not considering psychiatry at the beginning of medical school change their minds once they have clinical exposure to the specialty. Interestingly, a study by Lau et al. (2015) found that the amount of exposure to psychiatry in preclerkship years was associated with the chance students would declare for psychiatry, thus arguing further for earlier and more teaching of psychiatric ideas in medical school. Many medical students come to the profession because of the appeal of the patient–doctor relationship, the narratives of illness, and the power of connection, so it can be argued that experience with psychotherapy is especially well suited to inspire them to consider psychiatry.

Writing at a time when recruiting students into psychiatry was at a low, Herz (1984) argued that medical students needed more explicit instruction about and support for countertransference, lest they be alienated by their initial forays into psychiatry. It is important to normalize that psychiatry involves strong feelings—both the patient's and the therapist's—as well as many different kinds of identification with patients, all of which are used to deepen understanding of the patient and their mental suffering.

Strauss (1950) described a program for third-year medical students during their required clerkship in which the students observed four weekly sessions of an actual patient's new psychotherapy. At the conclusion of the four sessions, the patient was transferred to another clinician for ongoing therapeutic treatment. The instructor led the students in discussions focused on defining the patient's reasons for coming to therapy, their expectations of therapy, and their responses to psychodynamic interventions. Strauss noted that effort was made to stay close to the actual material and to avoid "wild conjectures" about the patient's unconscious. Anecdotally, the experience led to a decrease in distrustful attitudes toward psychiatry and an increasing interest in the profession on the part of the medical students (Strauss 1950).

Frank et al. (1987) described the impact of an outpatient site for the core clerkship in psychiatry at which students obtained clinical experience providing short-term psychotherapy. Patients were carefully selected: those with suicidality, psychosis, impulsivity, severe attachment disorders, and personality disorders were excluded. The patients agreed to a course of 10–12 sessions over 7 weeks of the 8-week clerkship. Supervision was quite intensive—5 hours/week as a group—and focused on developing themes, hearing conflicts in associations, transference, and countertransference. Compared with the other traditional clerkship sites, the outpatient site was more frequently requested and had higher satisfaction ratings on completion. In addition, the authors found a statistically significant increase in students selecting psychiatry as a career on follow-up (Frank et al. 1987).

Understanding Psychotherapy and Referring

There is no expectation that every doctor will treat mental health issues. Some aspects can be integrated into general internal medicine and family medicine practices, such as knowing when to refer a patient, and to what. Simply telling the patient they need a therapist is not helpful. Experience with psychotherapy during medical school may lead to a clearer understanding of what psychotherapy is, who may find it useful, and what a patient can expect from the treatment.

An eight-session course on psychodynamic psychotherapy was described by Ornstein (1961), consisting of a lecture on therapeutic principles, watching and discussing a recording of an actual session, role-playing, and a demonstration of hypnotically induced symptoms in a volunteer medical student resolved through a therapeutic interview. Ratings of the course were excellent, and the author's perception was that the most valuable impact was on reducing "literal-mindedness." Students gained an understanding that symptoms presenting to psychotherapy can be symbolically meaningful and that an exploratory approach to discovering concealed meaning can be valuable (Ornstein 1961).

Ball and Wolff (1963) described a program of medical students providing psychotherapy to selected patients under supervision. Their data were anecdotal, but their impression was that the patients did as well as they might have with experienced therapists because of the additional energy and attention the students brought to the task. They reported that students learned some foundational skills regarding the doctor–patient relationships and some familiarity with the principles of therapy, but the most valuable outcome was their appreciation that "psychotherapy proper is a highly complex method of treatment which can be mastered only by long and specialized training" (Ball and Wolff 1963, p. 216).

Cabaniss (1999) reflected on her experience of teaching clerkship students about the psychoanalytic process, noting that there can be some reluctance on the part of the students initially, "but psychoanalysts should be able to handle resistance" (p. 199). She believed that the seminar resulted in future physicians who would be better informed and therefore more effective at referring patients to therapy (Cabaniss 1999). Most recently, Aboul-Fotouh and Asghar-Ali (2010) reported that a resident-led elective course increased medical students' understanding of psychotherapy and the value of referral. The course comprised six hour-long sessions that used lecture, video clips, and role-play to teach the most common models of psychotherapy, including cognitive-behavioral therapy and supportive, interpersonal, and psychodynamic therapies. Student feedback also suggested that the course was useful in confirming attendees' interest in a psychiatric career (Aboul-Fotouh and Asghar-Ali 2010).

Enhancing Empathy

Longitudinal studies have shown a decrease in empathy over the course of medical school and residency. The reasons for this are myriad, but the fact remains that taking care of people requires an understanding of where they are coming from and what troubles they bring beside just a presenting problem. Effective empathy is part of being an effective doctor and, moreover, part of engaging with patients in their care. Neumann et al. (2011) found that this kind of understanding and communication with patients enhanced symptom reporting by the patient, diagnostic accuracy by the doctor, and satisfaction of the patient. Although some emotional empathy is innate, cognitive empathy can be taught and enhanced through attention, listening, and active efforts at getting in touch with the emotional responsiveness that helps us understand others. Empathy has been taught as part of simulated patient labs and exercises and leads to a decrease in the need to put distance between oneself and one's patient (Díez-Goñi and Rodríguez-Díez 2017). There have been arguments that this distance interferes with clinical care and robs physicians of their ability to join in addressing health care inequities and other issues (Holmes 2025). Psychotherapy may serve as a magnifying lens that increases the prominence and clarity of empathy in interpersonal encounters, and thus psychiatry educators have suggested that it may have value in empathetic development.

Philip et al. (2010) described a 1-hour module, "Crash Course in Supportive Psychotherapy," that they delivered to students in their core psychiatry clerkship. The module included didactic teaching, role-playing, and discussion and focused on improving empathetic response through a nonjudgmental stance and mobilizing hope. The authors reported that their pilot demonstrated that students enthusiastically received the instruction and felt better prepared for patient–physician communication. They additionally hoped that this experience would aid in recruitment into psychiatry (Philip et al. 2010).

Bender (2016) argued for the value of teaching psychodynamic thinking and principles to all medical students as a path toward increasing empathy. She described a two-session intervention during the required clerkship where she presented students with process notes from one of her own analytic cases and engaged them in active discussion about the value of her responses to the patients and their alternative suggestions. She humorously informed the students at the outset that they would all benefit from these lessons "unless they are going into pathology and have a dead patient" (Bender 2016).

Therapeutic Skills for Difficult Patients

Every doctor deals with a "difficult" patient at one point or another. Generally this term is used for a patient who does not cooperate in their care as expected or who evokes uncomfortable and unpleasant feelings in the physician. Such a patient, however, does not consciously intend to cause distress to or damage their relationship with a clinician. These outcomes are often the result of insufficient appreciation by the clinician that some aspect of psychopathology is driving the undesirable behaviors. The patient may have developed maladaptive coping patterns and defenses that are core to personality disorders and may also be triggered by the experience of anxiety, depression, psychosis, or addiction. This can in turn lead to high utilization of medical care, as well-intended interventions go awry, inappropriate interventions are sought, and patients move from clinician to clinician (Hahn et al. 1996). Learning basic therapeutic understanding and response to difficult patients helps disarm the situation and preserve the patient–doctor relationship.

McNeilly and Wengel (2001) created a clerkship seminar using the TV program "ER" to teach psychotherapeutic techniques relevant to the interview and management of patients with personality disorders (difficult patients). After viewing vignettes from the show, students were asked to reflect on their countertransference, articulate their own emotional reactions, and practice clarity of communication and setting boundaries. The authors found significant improvement in understanding of countertransference and knowledge of boundaries in pre- and postseminar tests of knowledge (McNeilly and Wengel 2001).

In a related report, Ghatavi and Waisman (2006) described a resident-led seminar for medical students that taught a psychotherapeutic approach to understanding and responding to people with personality disorders. The course used scenes from popular cinema and television series to illustrate pathology and engaged students in role-play to simulate the stresses of interactions with such patients. The course was rated highly by students, and the authors believed that it helped change their attitudes, moving from a view of "problem patients" to an examination of their own reactive feelings in the service of diagnostic formulation (Ghatavi and Waisman 2006).

What Should We Teach?

As the reader now appreciates, teaching psychotherapy has not been a single, unitary endeavor. Authors have described teaching different kinds of therapy with many different emphases regarding skills. However, evidence has shown that many of the common elements in all of these therapies are what motivate change and, therefore, may be what should be taught. Some of the techniques can be successfully taught across a range of specialties to incorporate into even the most time-crunched practices, ideas based in supportive therapy and cognitive behavioral therapy being chief among these (Truong et al. 2015).

Next, we discuss the content of the teaching of psychotherapeutic elements and what is of value for medical students to learn. Learning how to operationalize these techniques helps a doctor go into each patient encounter prepared to use them. We believe that medical students should learn a core set of psychotherapeutic skills grounded in the common elements of all psychotherapies. These include 1) feeling and communicating *empathy*; 2) setting *boundaries* for treatment; and 3) creating rapport and a treatment *alliance*.

Empathy

Empathy is a complex skill that involves affective, cognitive, and communicative components. Cognitive empathy is perhaps the most easily teachable, as it involves students learning to think their way into a patient's perspective. This can be taught in many ways including didactic lectures, case discussion, role-playing as patient, and video discussion formats. Students should recognize that they "think their way into" someone else's experience every time they watch a movie or a TV show and discuss with friends the characters' state of mind.

Patients often tell doctors how they are feeling in both verbal and nonverbal ways. Making note of body language, expression, and gaze helps the doctor discern what might be going on for the patient. Often a patient may not have the words for the emotions they are feeling, may be feeling too many or not enough emotions, or may be reacting in ways that suggest emotions under the surface of consciousness. Providing a shared language of the experience—how to speak to patients about this and name feelings they might be having—is crucial. We find it helpful to start with very basic kinds of experience and use the rubric that most patients we meet will be "mad, sad, or scared" (Rako and Mazer 1980,

p. 115). The educator can then build on this affective skeleton to illustrate the many different shades and nuances—and therefore distinct words—for the array of feelings that come under the umbrella of anger, sadness, and fear.

Medical students should also be taught that whatever else is going on with their patient, it is very possible that shame is involved. Shame is often underrecognized in both general medical settings and psychotherapy. It is valuable for students to appreciate how easily painful experiences and conditions can be made worse by an additional layering of shame.

Affective empathy (how we emotionally resonate with a patient's feelings) is of course hard to teach. It seems fair to say that people enter medical school with a spectrum of ability based on their temperament, and some may not be as in touch with this component as others. There are some things that the educator can do to help students tap into their capacities, however. First, talking to a patient about their distress will often evoke pain, as does palpating the abdomen of a patient with gastrointestinal complaints, and we should not shy away from this. It is not harmful for a patient to cry, nor is it harmful for a physician to become teary-eyed in response to their patient's suffering. In helping students become more in touch with their own capacity for affective resonance, once again film, TV, and popular music can be useful tools. Actors and singers are very skillful in evoking the viewer's or listener's feelings and drawing them into awareness. When we watch or listen together with students, we can help them identify their reactions to the artistic distillation of feelings.

We recommend instructing students to use simple techniques of leaning in and offering sympathetic facial expressions to convey that they are listening and that the patient is not alone with their feelings. Unfortunately, many patients today may go through entire visits where the doctor does not make eye contact with them, instead typing their clinic notes the entire time. We may need to help students relearn the power of face-to-face attention. Students should also learn some basic ways to help patients access feelings that remain unspoken, such as saying, "that sounds scary" or "that sounds very sad." These very simple interventions give relief to patients who feel anxious or overwhelmed in the face of a medical issue or diagnosis. Being supportive of a patient's experience by validating their feelings ("of course you felt…" or "other patients have said they felt…") can normalize the feeling state, empower the patient to explore further, and directly diminish shame.

Boundaries

We recommend that psychotherapy education for medical students focus on the concept of boundaries. Like empathy, boundaries are essential throughout all of medicine, and psychotherapy's distilled concentration of the patient–clinician relationship makes it the ideal laboratory for learning this topic. Students should learn that boundaries are not primarily a matter of ethical rules; rather, they are a way of structuring relationships to maximize a set of goals and minimize risks. Boundaries may be more fluid in different aspects of medicine. The primary goal of boundaries is to prevent exploitation of the patient and create a safe environment for them to discuss their care.

Privacy is of course the main boundary for physicians. The knowledge that their medical record and history are confidential and not being discussed in identifying ways outside of clinic allows a patient to discuss their presenting concern. Knowing that examination spaces and consultation areas are private and designed for that purpose allow patients to let down their defenses. Similarly, students should learn about the boundaries of personal space, such as what types of touch are necessary for examinations, what types are unwelcome, and what types are different depending on the type of doctor. A hospital-based internal medicine doctor might touch a patient on the arm to convey comfort or support in a tough time, whereas a clinic-based doctor might only shake hands and do necessary touching for a physical examination. Thinking about the ways in which touch can be interpreted and misinterpreted, and finding verbal ways to convey one's empathy and care, are important skills not only for psychiatrists but for all physicians. Discussing dual roles (such as friendships and work acquaintanceships with patients) and how to think about these roles is important. Additionally, chance meetings with patients outside of the work world (such as running into them at the store) should be addressed.

An important secondary benefit of boundaries is not only for the patient but for the doctor as well. Preventing burnout and work dissatisfaction often relies on the ability to know what you can and cannot heal, which worries and concerns can go home with you into your non-work world and which should remain at work. Boundaries allow the clinician, as a medical student and later as a physician, to bring their best possible self to their work.

Psychotherapy also provides an excellent vehicle for teaching students how to think about self-disclosure. For example, what is a patient entitled to know about the clinician (e.g., training status, nature of supervision) for the purposes of informed consent? What other kinds of self-disclosure may be requested by patients in their efforts to feel at ease, such as culture, religion, sexuality, marital status, and recovery status? We recommend explicit discussion with medical students about how such disclosures may increase comfort but simultaneously create confusion about boundaries.

Alliance

One of the most important things for medical students to learn is that there is a robust evidence base demonstrating that a strong therapeutic alliance, regardless of the specific type of therapy, is perhaps the best predictor of treatment success. We emphasize to students that a therapeutic alliance is founded on shared goals in an atmosphere of trust. The alliance communicates, "We have a common goal: to get you better." It is important to remind students to think about a patient's treatment goals, not just their own goals. Medical students are unlikely to appreciate without clear instruction that setting goals is always a negotiation that aims at a unified and integrated collaboration.

Students should learn the qualities that contribute to building an atmosphere of trust. These include transparency, confidentiality, tact, reliability, and respect for autonomy. *Transparency* means simply telling the patient the truth, with kindness and gentleness. Honesty and a "nothing-to-hide" presentation of facts saves the patient from worrying about any subterfuge going on in the room. *Confidentiality* allows a patient to open up, as best they can, about what symptoms they are having, even embarrassing ones. It allows them to ask questions, even when they're worried the question is "stupid." It protects from the feeling they are being criticized or mocked outside of the room or outside of the clinic.

The use of *tact* tends to create better outcomes, even when dealing with difficult patients or patients who are hearing difficult news. Being gentle with communication (as opposed to being gruff or blunt) may take more effort—but it does not take more time. In fact, helping students examine their approach to how they speak to patients ultimately saves them a great deal of time that is otherwise lost to unnecessary conflict and attempts at repair. *Reliability* is one of the more complicated pieces to achieve in the alliance. Myriad contact points—making appointments, getting in touch with the doctor, arriving on time, and refilling prescriptions—all lead to a sense that one's doctor is reliable.

Starting on time and ending on time in therapy is not just a boundary, it is a way of demonstrating the therapist's reliability. Reliability is similarly important in all patient–physician relationships. If you say you will put in for a test or submit a referral, then it should happen without the patient having to contact the office a second or third time.

Respect for autonomy is about respecting that a patient (or a patient's guardian) has the right to accept or refuse treatment. A doctor can advise, offer wisdom, and cite science to back up their recommendations, but at the end of the day the patient has the right to ignore that information. They have the right to get a second or third opinion, to seek alternative treatments the medical community might not recommend, and in many cases, to do so without interference from the medical community. A patient can be invited to participate in their care and their healing, but they cannot be forced to accept the invitation. This is especially clear when examining patients' decisions to begin or continue psychotherapy.

Some educators have recommended instruction that focuses on the formulation of maladaptive defenses and symbolic meaning in teaching medical students psychotherapy, especially with the aim of better understanding difficult patients. In our view, these are valuable elective topics for developing a more advanced understanding, but most difficult patients will respond to an approach that focuses on empathy, clear boundaries, and a focus on building trust and shared goals. For cases that do not respond, further instruction in formulating immature defenses or maladaptive cognitive schema is valuable.

Conclusions

Attempting to teach psychotherapy to medical students may initially seem overwhelming and unnecessary. Yet there are significant potential benefits to pursue. Recruiting into psychiatry may improve, the chance of effective future referrals may increase, decreases in empathy may be mitigated, and difficult patients may be more successfully engaged. We recommend that given the limited time available in both preclinical and clerkship curricula, a very focused approach to teaching psychotherapy is indicated, one that maximizes the concepts that have the greatest salience for a general physician and that are most clearly illuminated by the process of psychotherapy. Accordingly, we emphasize helping medical students learn how to deepen empathy, how to set boundaries according to underlying interests, and how to build alliances that rest on interpersonal trust and shared goals.

Key points

- Numerous potential benefits stem from exposing medical students to psychotherapy.
- Learning about psychotherapy has the potential to increase enthusiasm in a career in psychiatry.
- Learning about psychotherapy helps medical students understand the key elements of when and why to refer to psychiatry.
- Learning about psychotherapy increases empathy in medical students and provides benefits for both the patient and the doctor.
- Learning about psychotherapy teaches medical students how to work with difficult patients.
- Psychotherapy education should focus on common factors (such as empathy, boundaries, and alliance) that are widely relevant to all medical practice.

References

Aboul-Fotouh F, Asghar-Ali AA: Therapy 101: a psychotherapy curriculum for medical students. Acad Psychiatry 34(4):248–252, 2010 20576980

Ball DH, Wolff HH: An experiment in the teaching of psychotherapy to medical students. Lancet 1(7274):214–217, 1963 13966129

Bender EP: Teaching medical students psychodynamic psychotherapy: an interactive method. Acad Psychiatry 40(2):396–397, 2016 26768139

Cabaniss DL: How to think like an analyst 101: a model for teaching psychotherapy to medical students. J Psychother Pract Res 8(3):198–200, 1999 10413437

Díez-Goñi N, Rodríguez-Díez M: Why teaching empathy is important for the medical degree [in Spanish]. Rev Clin Esp 217(6):332–335, 2017

Frank D, Propst A, Goldhamer P: The effects of teaching medical students psychotherapy skills in the outpatient department. Can J Psychiatry 32(3):185–189, 1987 3567833

Freud S: On Psychotherapy, in Collected Papers Vol 1, Early Papers on the History of the Psycho-analytic Movement. Translated by Riviere J. New York, Basic Books, 1904; reprinted 1959, p 251

Ghatavi K, Waisman Z: Teaching medical students about personality disorders and psychotherapeutic principles: a resident pilot initiative. Acad Psychiatry 30(2):178–179, 2006 16609127

Hahn SR, Kroenke K, Spitzer RL, et al: The difficult patient: prevalence, psychopathology, and functional impairment. J Gen Intern Med 11(1):1–8, 1996 8691281

Herz LR: Aspects of teaching psychotherapy to medical students. Psychiatr Q 56(2):151–156, 1984 6531425

Holmes SM: Learning language, un/learning empathy in medical school. Cult Med Psychiatry 49(1):40–64, 2025 37725219

Lau T, Zamani D, Lee EK, et al: Factors affecting recruitment into psychiatry: a Canadian experience. Acad Psychiatry 39(3):246–252, 2015 25583402

McNeilly DP, Wengel SP: The "ER" seminar: teaching psychotherapeutic techniques to medical students. Acad Psychiatry 25(4):193–200, 2001 11744535

Neumann M, Edelhäuser F, Tauschel D, et al: Empathy decline and its reasons: a systematic review of studies with medical students and residents. Acad Med 86(8):996–1009, 2011 21670661

Ornstein PH: An experiment in teaching psychotherapy to junior medical students. J Med Educ 36(2):154–161, 1961 13731260

Philip NS, Rost-Banik D, Shaffer S, et al: Supportive psychotherapy: a crash course for medical students. Acad Psychiatry 34(1):57–60, 2010 20071730

Rako S, Mazer H (eds): Semrad: The Heart of a Therapist. New York, Jason Aronson, 1980

Satiani A, Niedermier J, Satiani B, Svendsen DP: Projected workforce of psychiatrists in the United States: a population analysis. Psychiatr Serv 69(6):710–713, 2018 29540118

Strauss BV: Teaching psychotherapy to medical students. J Assoc Am Med Coll 25(4):263–268, 1950 24537856

Substance Abuse and Mental Health Services Administration: Results from the 2017 National Survey on Drug Use and Health (NSDUH): key substance use and mental health indicators in the United States. Rockville, MD, Center for Behavioral Health Statistics and Quality. H-53, Publication No. SMA 18-5068, NSDUH Series, 2018. Available at: https://library.samhsa.gov/product/results-2017-national-survey-drug-use-and-health-nsduh-key-substance-use-and-mental-health. Accessed September 19, 2023.

Truong A, Wu P, Diez-Barroso R, Coverdale J: What is the efficacy of teaching psychotherapy to psychiatry residents and medical students? Acad Psychiatry 39(5):575–579, 2015 25933647

9

Education in Psychiatric Research for Medical Students

Marsal Sanches, M.D., Ph.D.
Michelle Patriquin, Ph.D.

The last several decades have witnessed a marked decline in the number of physician-scientists in the United States. Available data indicate that, compared with PhDs, physicians are less likely to be successful when initially applying for federal funds and to be awarded funds subsequently (Back et al. 2011). Consequently, the "triple-threat" academic physician, who successfully combines sound clinical work, excellence in education, and research expertise, is on the verge of extinction (Conti 1999). Research is in danger of becoming an extracurricular activity and not directly related to medical education curriculum (Kim et al. 2023).

Offering medical students research education has several potential benefits, but it becomes particularly critical considering the scenario above. Early exposure to research has been cited as a feasible way to identify potential future medical researchers, encourage students to engage in research-related activities, and provide guidance for those interested in pursuing a research-related career. Traditionally, research training in medical education has been relegated to a secondary place, although more recent numbers point to changes in that trend. In several medical schools around the world, research education for students seems to have become a priority, with specific curricula, faculty, and assistant deanships specifically dedicated to that aspect of medical education. Most generally, however, despite the importance of research and extracurricular activities in medical education (Kim et al. 2023), research has been defined as an "indirect" extracurricular activity or an activity that is "relatively unrelated to the student's major or curriculum" (Bartkus et al. 2012, p. 699; Kim et al. 2023).

This chapter contains an overview of undergraduate medical research education, particularly psychiatric research. First, we cover the potential benefits and the current status of research education for undergraduate medical students, followed by challenges and obstacles sometimes faced while implementing undergraduate medical research education initiatives. Next, we outline practical aspects and interventions of interest in research education for undergraduate medical students. Last, we discuss some of the future perspectives in medical student training and education in the particular field of psychiatry research.

Why Research Education for Medical Students?

Available evidence supports that research education for undergraduate medical students helps build a solid scientific foundation for future physicians. For example, attendance at a research methodology course positively affects medical students' attitudes toward science in medicine (Vujaklija et al. 2010). Still, many undergraduate medical students demonstrate limited knowledge regarding research and its importance for their training as future physicians (El Achi et al. 2020; Vodopivec et al. 2002). Moreover, in a 2016 study, fewer than half of undergraduate medical students reported believing their medical schools provided enough opportunities for students to engage in research activities (Funston et al. 2016).

There are several potential benefits in providing medical students with experiences in psychiatric research education, even for students not primarily interested in an academic career. This experience helps reduce the gap between basic science and clinical practice, which has become a topic of particular importance as psychiatry has become progressively more scientific and much closer to neuroscience in terms of its foundations, including its conceptual, diagnostic, and clinical aspects (Sanches 2024). Therefore, a solid basis in research may help medical students develop more scientifically oriented decision-making abilities regarding practical clinical aspects of psychiatry, reducing the risk of diagnostic biases and other heuristics during clinical decision-making.

In addition, research education for undergraduate medical students may increase the physician-scientist pipeline. Research engagement at an undergraduate level makes medical students more aware of possible research careers, helps students identify specific areas of research interest, enhances students' research efficacy and academic performance, increases intention to pursue academic work, and allows mentors to identify trainees with particular talent for research (DiBiase et al. 2020; Ommering et al. 2021). Retrospective studies indicate that medical students who participated in research programs during their undergraduate training seemed more likely to remain scientifically active, publish more, and occupy academic positions after graduation (Radville et al. 2019).

Unfortunately, there is no true consensus about the impact of such educational interventions. At least one prospective study indicated that the implementation of an extracurricular research program for medical students, while having positive effects on academic achievement and motivation for research, did not produce statistically significant effects on research self-efficacy beliefs, curiosity, or perceptions of research (Ommering et al. 2021) after an 18-month follow-up period. It is not yet clear what baseline factors predict a better outcome in cultivating interest in research and nurturing future research scientists. These results point to the need for studies that characterize the profile of students more likely to benefit from research education interventions.

In psychiatric education specifically, research training may have an additional role in helping consolidate scientific psychiatry among medical students. Despite its well-established place as a medical specialty, psychiatry is often still mistakenly perceived by students as excessively subjective, ineffective in terms of treatment, and wed to psychoanalytical concepts, many of which are difficult to quantify. Research education might produce a positive impact on the attitude of medical students toward psychiatry and help them develop critical and analytical skills related to the diagnostic process in psychiatry, the validity and reliability of adopted diagnostic categories, the impact of treatments in terms of risks versus benefits, and a better characterization of outcomes in psychiatric care.

Practical Aspects of Research Education for Undergraduate Medical Students

Over the past several years, different medical schools worldwide have implemented research-focused scholar programs for medical students. Some are incorporated into the required medical school curriculum, and others are extracurricular research opportunities. The names of these extracurricular options vary significantly: research electives, summer research programs, and scholar programs, for example. In addition, many students take the initiative (or receive invitations) to become informally involved in research conducted by faculty members. This informal involvement in research may take place in different forms, depending on the student's interest, background, and time availability and the needs of the faculty mentor, and can include benchwork, data collection, literature review, data analysis, and drafting of scientific manuscripts.

Intracurricular Research Education

The rationale for including a research education component in the medical school mandatory curriculum is simple: many medical students express interest in becoming proficient in research, but few become involved, partly because of limited opportunities. Several medical schools have incorporated research education components into their curricula, but the intensity of these components varies significantly. Research education is sometimes limited to lectures and theoretical discussions surrounding basic concepts and scientific methodology. In other cases, students are required to develop a specific research project under the guidance of a faculty member and become acquainted with different practical aspects of research.

In one example of such an approach, students took a required "research practicum." They were exposed to the logistics of research at different phases, including critically analyzing literature, formulating research questions and hypothesis, conducting a literature review, choosing and implementing the most appropriate research approach, documenting and interpreting results, and exploring research-related ethical issues (Jacobs and Costin 2022). According to available evidence, students' satisfaction and productivity levels are similar for such mandatory research involvement during medical school as for elective research rotations (Chang and Ramnanan 2015). Such findings argue in favor of expanding the inclusion of research education as part of the mandatory medical school curriculum.

Nevertheless, including formal psychiatric research education elements in the psychiatry medical school curriculum may be challenging because of the constant expansion of the mandatory components and disciplines covered during medical school and the limited amount of time allocated to teaching certain areas and specialties, including psychiatry. In many cases, research education is introduced under the umbrella of evidence-based teaching and included in the curriculum using a matrix-like approach across different modules and subjects. In some medical schools, students are required to complete a formal research project under the guidance of a faculty mentor but are given latitude as to the topic and area of concentration of the project in question, allowing those with a specific interest in psychiatry to focus their projects in that direction.

There are concerns about the potential adverse effects of intense research education at an undergraduate medical education level. Given the absence of definitive data regarding the full impact of research education in terms of improving patient care and increasing interest in academic careers among students, the potential benefits of mandatory research need to be balanced against other factors, such as financial implications, availability of faculty mentors, and impact on the school's educational culture (Parsonnet et al. 2010). In one survey of 558 medical students, 70% expressed interest in participating in research activities during medical school, but only 26% supported making research training a mandatory part of the medical school curriculum (Park et al. 2010).

Research Electives

Research electives represent an alternative (or, at times, a complement) to intracurricular research education interventions. Medical schools can offer research electives as an option for medical students to fulfill their elective time, usually during their junior or senior year. Depending on the institution in question, structured, pre-approved electives (with well-delineated components, requirements, and expectations) are available, usually within specific areas and specialties. In other instances, an elective can be individually tailored and designed on a case-by-case basis according to the student's interests and the availability of faculty mentors. The duration of research electives may vary widely, from 2–4 weeks to 3 months. In the case of highly competitive research electives, selection criteria also differ from program to program. Some schools prioritize a record of previous research experience and an academic portfolio pointing to a specific interest in a physician-scientist career. Available literature supports the positive impact of medical school research electives on nurturing future research careers. In one study, medical school graduates who completed research electives with scientific writing/authorship experience were more likely to subsequently be awarded extramural research funds, including F32, mentored-K, and R01 awards (Jeffe and Andriole 2018).

Given their nonmandatory nature, research electives are more likely to attract students with previous research experience or particular interest in a research or academic career, so it is hard to generalize their benefits for students overall. Research electives will compete with clinical electives, which will be more attractive for students primarily interested in a nonacademic career. In one study, only one-third of surveyed medical students expressed interest in enrolling in a formal 12-week research elective, although more than 70% of the participants did report some involvement in research during their undergraduate medical training (Pheley et al. 2006). The authors also reported that students' interest in electives was twice as high when clinical or population-based research was considered, as opposed to basic research.

Moreover, it is our experience that achieving a final research product (e.g., in the form of a paper submission, a letter to the editor, or a poster presentation) as a result of the time spent in electives is a strong motivator for medical students. Such tangible results may pave the way for further involvement in research and help students obtain financial aid to attend scientific conferences. Given the limited amount of time allocated to research electives, however, it may not be feasible for students to complete a research project involving original data collection. One alternative is to work with medical students to analyze previously collected data, helping them formulate research questions and specific hypotheses and test them using available datasets. In those cases, the adequate matching between research elective students and faculty members becomes crucial.

Despite the apparent straightforward goals for a research elective, the core competencies learned can be formulated in different ways and often transcend the field of medical research. For example, involvement in an overseas early research elective may represent a valuable opportunity to foster international collaborations and help students develop resilience, adaptability, creativity, and familiarity with multiculturalism (Dawidziuk et al. 2020). Preparing students to deal with uncertainty, an essential skill for virtually any physician, could be one of the main benefits of attending such research electives.

The research literature on undergraduate psychiatry research electives is minimal. The authors have previoulsy implemented a full-time, 4-week research elective for medical students. In addition to acquiring hands-on research experience with data analysis and scientific writing, students attend research meetings (e.g., journal club sessions), participate in research participant assessments, and complete a cycle of seminars focusing on basic aspects of medical research (Table 9.1). Although previous experience with research is not necessary, students with a research background are more likely to take full advantage of the research rotation. Students are evaluated by their faculty mentors on a pass/fail grading system. Teachers evaluate active participation in research-related activities, attendance of didactic seminars, and completion of at least one acceptable scholarly poster presentation or scientific paper.

Summer Research Initiatives

Summer research initiatives may represent an alternative to formal electives for students interested in becoming involved in research during medical school. The formats may differ regarding the program's frequency, duration, and purpose. In some cases, summer research programs are independent, single periods of research work between school years. In other cases, participating students are selected at the beginning of medical school and offered continued summer research

Table 9.1 Topics on medical research covered during a psychiatry research elective

Study designs: how to choose the proper study
Critical analysis of scientific papers
Systematic reviews and meta-analysis
How to prepare a letter to the editor
Writing a case report
Career advice for prospective physician-scientists
Scientific misconduct

experiences over their undergraduate medical training under the guidance of the same mentor. Certain summer research programs offer benefits to selected participants, including housing and stipends, and often require presentation of a conclusion project.

Summer research programs can be highly competitive and frequently vary in scope. In some institutions, such programs are available for internal undergraduate medical students; in others, they are not directed to medical students but to undergraduate college students attending pre–health professions tracks or, in some cases, to high school students. Some available summer school programs specifically aim to increase research opportunities for underrepresented minorities (Schwartz et al. 2022). In one instance, medical students from underrepresented minorities were selected for a virtual summer program that included pairing with a mentor, joining virtual meetings, working on core research projects, and preparing an oral presentation (Masaki et al. 2022).

Given the usually short duration of summer research programs, their primary goal is to enhance students' interest in the field of research; data support the notion that they are effective in achieving that goal. In one study, for example, 75% of participants in an undergraduate medical school summer research program reported increased research interest. Fully 85% of the participants stated that the program was effective in helping them understand research methodology and expressed intent to continue incorporating research in their medical careers (Cain et al. 2019).

Additionally, available evidence does suggest that such programs can have positive effects on increasing student's research self-efficacy. One study (Black et al. 2013) combined and analyzed data from three separate National Institutes of Health–funded summer research programs, including the Medical Students' Sustained Training and Research Experience in Aging and Mental Health, a single-site summer research initiative focused on geriatric psychiatry or neuroscience research (Jeste et al. 2018). Results indicated improvements in students' overall perceived self-efficacy for research, particularly regarding their understanding of research methodology and communication (Black et al. 2013).

Scientific Publishing

Although feedback from medical students might suggest that the emphasis of research opportunities for medical students should be placed on the learning process instead of the output (Mabvuure 2012), research findings indicate that medical students whose research involvement resulted in publication before graduation are more likely to subsequently remain engaged with scientific activities, including a higher likelihood to continue to publish and to achieve higher citation impact (Waaijer et al. 2019). Nevertheless, only a minority of medical students in research training programs translate their experience into publications. In one study, only 26% of medical students who attended summer research programs, and 25% of those completing a research elective at the same institution, produced publications (Parker et al. 2021).

Given these low publication rates among trainees, we need a better understanding of the elements associated with higher versus lower publication achievement. Curiously, in the same study just mentioned (Parker et al. 2021), factors associated with achieving publication differed between students who took summer research programs versus electives. Student-related factors (such as having attended a higher-ranked college or showing higher academic performance, as estimated by future Alpha Omega Alpha membership) seemed to be strongly associated with achieving publication during summer research programs. Mentor-related factors (having a doctorate, not having a doctor of medicine or osteopathy degree, and successfully publishing with prior mentees) were also associated with higher chances of publication among students who completed research electives. Contrary to the idea that mentoring students without previous publication experience may be particularly challenging and that such students are less likely to achieve publication, the study found that students' prior publication history was not associated with publication rates.

Evidence also suggests that sociodemographic inequalities are related to research productivity among medical students. In a multisite cross-sectional study in the United Kingdom (Osunronbi et al. 2023) involving data from 36 medical schools, women were less likely than men to have publications or be first author on publications. Compared with White students, students of mixed ethnicity were more likely to have publications and had a higher number of publications. In addition, students who attended private high schools, compared with public schools, were found to have higher rates of publication as first author.

Mentorship

A crucial aspect of research education for medical students involves the availability of proper mentorship. Some authors have emphasized the invaluable role of including students in research groups, given their enthusiasm, motivation, and up-to-date medical knowledge (Liddell and Heuertz 2011). In one study, authors who worked with medical students had a higher scholarly impact than those who worked only with physicians and doctoral-level researchers (Svider et al. 2014).

Nevertheless, mentoring research medical students, while seen by many as rewarding, may involve particular challenges, most related to limited funding and lack of protected time for mentorship. From an institutional standpoint, research mentorship involves key domains, each of which may involve certain institutional aspects for successful implementation (Keyser et al. 2008). Those include factors involved in the selection and motivation of mentors, factors influencing the relationship between mentors and mentees, elements that enhance the mentee's ability to perform research, and the professional development of both mentors and mentees (Table 9.2).

Practically speaking, research mentors are assigned according to their research experience, availability, and interest in mentoring medical students. An ideal mentor–mentee relationship needs to ensure personal growth by offering the student not only support but also challenges. The research mentor role often overlaps with the role of a teacher, coach, and sponsor (Beck Dallaghan et al. 2022). Because the background and level of familiarity with formal aspects of research varies widely among medical students, an adequate match between students and mentors is of high importance, especially regarding expectations. A poor fit between mentor and mentee is a commonly cited barrier to successful mentorship processes (Sambunjak et al. 2006). Competition between mentors and mentees is not uncommon, especially when the mentee seems to surpass their assigned mentor in their area of expertise; thus faculty humility is an essential feature for those mentoring medical students in research (Beck Dallaghan et al. 2022). A recent study focusing on the impact of research mentorship among prospective radiation oncology trainees during medical school indicated that students working with radiation oncology mentors are more likely to publish in oncology-oriented journals (Bono et al. 2023). Despite the absence of similar data in the field of psychiatry, these results suggest that assigned mentors' specialties and areas of expertise play a role in students' accomplishments and productivity associated with mentorship activities.

Last, regarding the impact of mentorship on trainees, data support the notion that formal mentorship programs are likely to positively affect the choice of psychiatry as a medical specialty among medical

Table 9.2 The five key domains of research mentorship

Criteria for mentor selection
Incentives for motivating faculty to work as mentors
Facilitating the mentor–mentee relationship
Strengthening the mentee's ability to conduct research properly
Professional development of mentees and mentors

Source. Adapted from Keyser et al. (2008).

students. For example, a recent study demonstrated that schools participating in mentorship programs sponsored by the Klingenstein Third Generation Foundation (which aims at increasing interest, awareness, and opportunities for clinical experience, advocacy, networking, and research in the field of child psychiatry) showed higher match rates into psychiatry compared with nonparticipating schools (Himmelstein et al. 2022). Other authors have proposed, however, that the short duration of research training opportunities for medical students might limit their impact in terms of career decisions (Roane et al. 2009). Additional research is needed on the long-term impact of mentorship among students considering psychiatry as a medical specialty.

Conclusions

Research education for medical students seems intuitively recommended, but there is no complete consensus regarding its different potential implications at individual and institutional levels. Given that such initiatives may involve extra costs and often require deviating faculty from clinical and other education roles, better clarity regarding the goals, structure, and necessary level of commitment of students and faculty involved in research mentorship seems essential. From a practical standpoint, based on our experience as medical educators, we regard specific points as particularly critical.

First, for students interested in research, we consider it essential to offer them a "happy" research experience. That includes realistic expectations considering the available time of both students and mentors and open negotiation regarding the student's primary research project, taking into account the student's interests, the mentor's expertise, and the nature and feasibility of the proposed project.

Second, despite concerns raised in the literature about undergraduate medical research programs being of limited quality, we believe that they should focus more on the process than the final outcome. Even so, the existence of a final research product makes the research education experience tangible and offers students and participating faculty a concrete addition to their portfolio. Therefore, we highly recommend aiming at a final research product in the form of a paper, a letter to the editor, a research abstract, or a poster presentation.

Third, we strongly support institutional efforts toward recognizing faculty research mentorship, not only from a funding and protected-time point of view but also through formal acknowledgment of such activities for purposes of promotion and tenure. Research education and mentorship involvement are promising yet relatively unexplored niches in faculty development.

Key Points

- Research education for medical students helps build a solid scientific foundation for future physicians, in addition to having a putative impact on increasing the physician-scientist pipeline. Specifically regarding psychiatric education, research training may help consolidate the concept of scientific psychiatry among medical students.
- A large variety of educational interventions, including curricular and extracurricular rotations, may be implemented to offer students a "happy" research experience, with realistic goals that consider students' individual interests and specific institutional factors.
- Additional research is needed to better clarify the full impact of research educational interventions for medical students and identify individual features associated with benefits from such interventions among students.

References

Back SE, Book SW, Santos AB, Brady KT: Training physician-scientists: a model for integrating research into psychiatric residency. Acad Psychiatry 35(1):40–45, 2011 21209406

Bartkus KR, Nemelka B, Nemelka M, Gardner P: Clarifying the meaning of extracurricular activity: a literature review of definitions (AJBE). Am J Bus Educ 5(6):693–704, 2012

Beck Dallaghan GL, Coe CL, Wright ST, Jordan SG: Mentoring medical education research: guidelines from a narrative review. Med Sci Educ 32(3):723–731, 2022 35818612

Black ML, Curran MC, Golshan S, et al: Summer research training for medical students: impact on research self-efficacy. Clin Transl Sci 6(6):487–489, 2013 24330695

Bono K, Palmeri M, Huang A, et al: Assessment of medical student research mentorship in radiation oncology. Adv Radiat Oncol 9(1):101323, 2023 38260215

Cain L, Kramer G, Ferguson M: The Medical Student Summer Research Program at the University of Texas Medical Branch at Galveston: building research foundations. Med Educ Online 24(1):1581523, 2019 30831061

Chang Y, Ramnanan CJ: A review of literature on medical students and scholarly research: experiences, attitudes, and outcomes. Acad Med 90(8):1162–1173, 2015 25853690

Conti CR: Can the triple-threat academic physician exist in the new millennium? Clin Cardiol 22(8):499, 1999 10576954

Dawidziuk A, Gandhewar R, Kulkarni Y: Early years research elective: changing perspectives and dealing with uncertainty. J Med Educ Curric Dev 7(January):2382120520965999, 2020 33225068

DiBiase RM, Beach MC, Carrese JA, et al: A medical student scholarly concentrations program: scholarly self-efficacy and impact on future research activities. Med Educ Online 25(1):1786210, 2020 32589550

El Achi D, Al Hakim L, Makki M, et al: Perception, attitude, practice and barriers towards medical research among undergraduate students. BMC Med Educ 20(1):195, 2020 32552801

Funston G, Piper RJ, Connell C, et al: Medical student perceptions of research and research-orientated careers: an international questionnaire study. Med Teach 38(10):1041–1048, 2016 27008336

Himmelstein R, Guth S, Enenbach M, et al: Psychiatry match rates increase after exposure to a medical student mentorship program: a multisite retrospective cohort analysis. Acad Psychiatry 46(1):40–44, 2022 32100255

Jacobs RJ, Costin J: A fully online research practicum curriculum for undergraduate medical students: a protocol paper. Cureus 14(11):e31901, 2022

Jeffe DB, Andriole DA: Prevalence and predictors of US medical graduates' federal F32, mentored-K, and R01 awards: a national cohort study. J Investig Med 66(2):340–350, 2018 28954846

Jeste DV, Avanzino J, Depp CA, et al: Effect of short-term research training programs on medical students' attitudes toward aging. Gerontol Geriatr Educ 39(2):214–222, 2018 28614041

Keyser DJ, Lakoski JM, Lara-Cinisomo S, et al: Advancing institutional efforts to support research mentorship: a conceptual framework and self-assessment tool. Acad Med 83(3):217–225, 2008 18316865

Kim S, Jeong H, Cho H, Yu J: Extracurricular activities in medical education: an integrative literature review. BMC Med Educ 23(1):278, 2023 37087451

Liddell PW, Heuertz RM: Students as vital participants in research projects. Clin Lab Sci 24(2):66–70, 2011 21657137

Mabvuure NT: Twelve tips for introducing students to research and publishing: a medical student's perspective. Med Teach 34(9):705–709, 2012 22905656

Masaki CO, Ogbu-Nwobodo L, Santos LH, et al: A virtual summer research and mentorship program for Underrepresented in Medicine (URiM) medical students in psychiatry. Acad Psychiatry 46(4):537–539, 2022 35414163

Ommering BWC, Van Blankenstein FM, Dekker FW: First steps in the physician-scientist pipeline: a longitudinal study to examine the effects of an undergraduate extracurricular research programme. BMJ Open 11(9):e048550, 2021

Osunronbi T, Adeboye W, Faluyi D, et al; REMED-U.K. collaborators: Predictors of self-reported research productivity amongst medical students in the United Kingdom: a national cross-sectional survey. BMC Med Educ 23(1):412, 2023 37280642

Park SJK, McGhee CNJ, Sherwin T: Medical students' attitudes towards research and a career in research: an Auckland, New Zealand study. N Z Med J 123(1323):34–42, 2010

Parker SM, Vona-Davis LC, Mattes MD: Factors predictive of publication among medical students participating in school-sponsored research programs. Cureus 13(9):e18176, 2021

Parsonnet J, Gruppuso PA, Kanter SL, Boninger M: Required vs. elective research and in-depth scholarship programs in the medical student curriculum. Acad Med 85(3):405–408, 2010 20182112

Pheley AM, Lois H, Strobl J: Interests in research electives among osteopathic medical students. J Am Osteopath Assoc 106(11):667–670, 2006 17192455

Radville L, Aldous A, Arnold J, Hall AK: Outcomes from an elective medical student Research Scholarly Concentration program. J Investig Med 67(6):1018–1023, 2019 30723119

Roane DM, Inan E, Haeri S, Galynker II: Ensuring research competency in psychiatric residency training. Acad Psychiatry 33(3):215–220, 2009 19574518

Sambunjak D, Straus SE, Marusić A: Mentoring in academic medicine: a systematic review. JAMA 296(9):1103–1115, 2006 16954490

Sanches M: Research education in psychiatry: luxury or necessity? Alpha Psychiatry 25(1):120–121, 2024 38799497

Schwartz L, Luban N, Hall A, et al: The mentored experience to enhance opportunities in research (METEOR) program. Med Educ Online 27(1):2014290, 2022 34878968

Svider PF, Husain Q, Mauro KM, et al: Impact of mentoring medical students on scholarly productivity. Int Forum Allergy Rhinol 4(2):138–142, 2014 24243770

Vodopivec I, Vujaklija A, Hrabak M, et al: Knowledge about and attitude towards science of first year medical students. Croat Med J 43(1):58–62, 2002 11828562

Vujaklija A, Hren D, Sambunjak D, et al: Can teaching research methodology influence students' attitude toward science? Cohort study and nonrandomized trial in a single medical school. J Investig Med 58(2):282–286, 2010 20130460

Waaijer CJF, Ommering BWC, van der Wurff LJ, et al; NVMO Special Interest Group on Scientific Education: Scientific activity by medical students: the relationship between academic publishing during medical school and publication careers after graduation. Perspect Med Educ 8(4):223–229, 2019 31290118

10

Assessment and Feedback to Medical Students During Psychiatry Rotations

Joshua A. Trull, D.O.
Allen C. Richert Jr., M.D.

The term *assessment* appears frequently in education literature, but a straightforward definition does not. There seems to be consensus that the process of assessment should 1) provide information about student progress toward achieving the objectives of an academic program and 2) create an opportunity for the student to receive feedback. *Feedback* refers to the act of giving the student information (typically obtained by assessment) about their performance to help them improve and advance along the pathway to achieving the educational outcomes of the program. The sophistication of assessment and feedback has evolved and will probably continue to evolve, but it is unlikely that their importance in education will diminish anytime soon. This chapter reviews the key aspects of assessment and feedback in the psychiatry clerkship.

Assessment

What Is Assessment?

Assessment is "the action ... of making a judgment about something" (Merriam-Webster 2025). The essential judgment that educators must make is the determination of medical student competence. The Liaison Committee on Medical Education (LCME) definition of assessment captures this concept: "the systematic use of a variety of methods to collect, analyze, and use information to determine whether a medical student has acquired the competencies that the profession and the public expect of a physician" (Liaison Committee on Medical Education 2023, p. 21). Young et al. (2021, p. 318) provided a helpful definition from the perspective of a medical educator, describing assessment as "the measurement (or gathering of information) of how a trainee performs on a given task (e.g., multiple choice question examination) to make inferences about their competence (e.g. medical knowledge about psychiatric illness)."

Assessment provides a method of determining whether a student has reached some predefined level of performance that will earn them the right to advance to the next level of training or licensure to practice (Cooke et al. 2010). It also provides a data set with which educators can make decisions regarding competency.

Feedback is an important component of assessment. The criteria of Norcini et al. (2011, p. 206) for good assessment state that assessment involves "testing, measuring, collecting, and combining information, and providing feedback." Feedback enables students to guide or focus their learning efforts (Cooke et al. 2010). The terms *summative* and *formative* distinguish between assessments performed for the ranking of students versus the provision of feedback. The adjective *formative* identifies assessments performed to facilitate learning. The adjective *summative* identifies assessments performed to determine success or achievement of some goal. Data provided by any assessment tool can be used for either formative or summative purposes, but some tools function better for one or the other purpose. Formative evaluations typically occur before the end of the course or rotation (e.g., midrotation assessments). The formative assessment identifies the strengths and weaknesses of the student's performance and provides meaningful data for constructive feedback designed to help the student achieve the objectives and competencies of the rotation. Summative assessments typically occur at the end of rotations or training. Examples of summative (sometimes referred to as "high-stakes") assessments include final examinations or licensing or certification examinations.

Despite decades of calls for change, assessment in medical education has traditionally consisted of summative assessments with multiple choice questions (MCQs) or objective structured clinical examinations (OSCEs). MCQ tests probe student knowledge—or, stated differently, what the student knows. Miller (1990, p. S63) suggested that "if we really believe there is more to the practice of medicine than knowing," then tests of knowledge, although important, are incomplete forms of assessment. To highlight the importance of assessing more than knowledge, Miller suggested a framework for clinical assessment (i.e., Miller's pyramid) that organizes aspects of competence into a hierarchy: 1) knowledge (what the student *Knows*), 2) competence (if the student *Knows How* to use his knowledge), 3) performance (the student *Shows How*), and 4) action (the student *Does* or employs his skill and knowledge in clinical situations). The competency-based medical education (CBME) movement of the early 2000s emphasized the attainment of abilities (or competencies) over memorization of long lists of knowledge objectives and time-based training requirements. CBME programs organize their curricula around competencies, which, in the context of CBME, are abilities or capabilities and may be viewed as "ingredients of competence" (Frank et al. 2010, p. 641).

Central to the CBME paradigm are the tenets that competence is multidimensional (i.e., involves multiple domains), is developmental (i.e., ability in a domain can range from novice to master [Dreyfus 2004]), and changes with time and context (Frank et al. 2010). CBME is organized around the question, What abilities are needed of graduates? (Harden et al. 1999). A curriculum based on competencies, therefore, "begins with outcomes in mind, on the basis of which it defines the abilities needed by graduates and then develops milestones, instructional methods, and assessment tools to facilitate their acquisition by learners" (Frank et al. 2010, p. 641). Of note, Frank et al. referred to assessments as tools to measure progress along the milestones.

Young et al. (2021) described the innovation of *workplace-based assessment* (WBA):

> In the competency-based era of outcomes-based education, the focus of assessment has shifted to the workplace domain of doing, what the trainee actually does in practice. This led to a new approach to assessment called workplace-based assessment. (p. 318)

The Accreditation Council for Graduate Medical Education (ACGME) Milestones Project and the AAMC Core Entrustable Professional

Activities (EPAs) both necessitate the use of WBAs. While WBA provides an obvious and theoretically gratifying approach to assess clinical competence, educator and trainee uncertainty about the educational benefits of WBAs and the difficulties of fitting them into busy work schedules have frustrated efforts to deploy assessment into the workplace (Cheung et al. 2019; Massie and Ali 2016).

Criteria or frameworks for good assessment can guide educators looking for available tools or developing their own. Norcini et al. (2018) described the characteristics of good assessment tools:

1. Validity or coherence: Research demonstrates and students and educators believe that the assessment measures the quality that it purports to measure.
2. Reproducibility, reliability, or consistency: Repeating the assessment in similar circumstances generates the same results.
3. Equivalence: Use of the asssessment at different institutions produces similar results.
4. Feasibility: It is practical to administer the assessment within its intended environment.
5. Educational effect: The assessment improves student attainment of the educational program's learning objectives.
6. Catalytic effect: The assessment motivates student effort to improve performance and educator effort to improve the educational program.
7. Acceptability: Educators and students can tolerate the assessment, and they believe in the usefulness of the assessment.

Norcini's criteria can help guide 1) selection of the optimum assessment for each situation and 2) development of new (better) assessments for those situations in which current assessment tools do not fit well.

The clerkship director need not be expert in assessment; however, they must be able to 1) select or develop assessment tools capable of measuring student attainment of the course objectives, 2) master (and teach others) the use of the clerkship assessments and any assessments that medical school requires, 3) ensure that students receive formative assessments in a supportive environment that catalyzes or stimulates learning, and 4) provide expert assessments in the domains of interpersonal communication and professionalism.

Before we review available assessment tools, it is important to acknowledge that no single assessment provides a reliable and valid determination of medical education competencies. The demonstration of student competence in a single domain requires the use of multiple assessments performed repeatedly during the educational program.

Assessment Tools

The ACGME Assessment Guidebook provides a list of medical education assessment tools and their characteristics (Holmboe and Iobst 2020). Even though the toolbox was designed for graduate medical education purposes, the assessments work in the context of undergraduate medical education. The assessment tools listed below are a sample of assessments listed in the ACGME Assessment Guidebook:

1. Standardized multiple choice question tests
2. Clinical questioning
3. Chart-stimulated recall
4. Assessment-of-reasoning tool
5. Faculty assessments, including global assessments
6. Clinical performance or record review
7. Simulation
8. Standardized (simulated) patients (OSCEs)
9. Direct observation
10. Multisource feedback (360 Feedback)

Standardized MCQ tests, such as the National Board of Medical Examiners (NBME) subject examinations and the U.S. Medical Licensing Examination (USMLE), are integral components of student assessment. They are convenient and effective for assessing the acquisition of medical knowledge. The MCQ has more research supporting its reliability and validity than any other assessment method. Its shortcomings include its cost and that it assesses only the lowest level of competence in Miller's pyramid, the *Knows* level (Miller 1990). Medical knowledge is important—it is the foundation on which competence is built—but the MCQ test alone is not a sufficient means of determining medical competence.

Clinical questioning probes both a student's acquired medical knowledge and their ability to apply that knowledge in the provision of clinical care. It is one step up on Miller's pyramid, *Knows how.* If an educator were to question one student at a time, it would not be time efficient, and capturing the competency data from clinical questioning is complicated. Clinical questioning can be performed in non-work-based, simulated, and work-based settings (e.g., rounding, morning reports, morbidity and mortality presentations, chart audits). Structured methods of clinical questioning include One-minute preceptor, Think aloud, and SNAPPS. One-minute preceptor divides the teaching process into five microskills: 1) encourage the student to commit to an answer; 2) probe for evidence to support their answer; 3) teach general rules; 4) reinforce what the student got right; and 5) correct the student's mistakes. This technique works in many settings and situations. An example of employing this technique to assess a student who participated in an initial outpatient evaluation might involve the preceptor 1) requiring the student to declare which DSM diagnosis best captures the patient's presentation, 2) asking the student what signs and symptoms in the patient's presentation led them to that diagnosis, 3) reviewing the criteria related to the diagnosis in question, 4) pointing out to the student which criteria they correctly identified, and 5) pointing out to the student which criteria they did not identify or erroneously included in their response. The Think aloud approach encourages the student to verbalize their reasoning as they think through a case. An example of a student using the technique properly should include statements such as, "Because the patient described feeling sad, has lost their appetite, and no longer gets joy from life, I suspect the diagnosis is major depressive disorder." SNAPPS (a mnemonic for summarize, narrow, analyze, probe, plan, and select) provides a structure for an educational encounter led by the student and facilitated by the preceptor in which the student presents a condensed medical history to allow time for the student to verbalize their thinking and reasoning. The validity and reliability of these clinical questioning methods vary. Planning where and how the assessments will be used, training faculty how to use them (including agreeing on what success looks like), and making students aware of the assessments tend to improve validity and reliability of clinical questioning.

Chart-stimulated recall (CSR) is a "chart review of a patient encounter with a structured oral examination" (Holmboe and Iobst 2020, p. 14) (a simple chart audit does not include the structured oral examination). The oral examination component of CSR can probe many aspects of the learner's clinical reasoning. Some aspects of professionalism and practice-based learning and improvement can be assessed with the addition of prompted self-assessment and reflective questioning. Note that CSR is considered a work-based assessment tool. Meaningful administration of CSR requires planned dedication of 30–60 minutes and education of faculty and learners before performing the assessment. CSR can provide assessments of clinical reasoning that are valid and reliable enough that the American Board of Emergency Medicine has used them to inform summative decisions regarding board certification. Note that CSR requires significant faculty training.

The Assessment of Reasoning Tool (ART) (by the Society to Improve Clinical Reasoning in Medicine) provides a structure for assessing clinical reasoning skills and benchmarks for minimal, partial, and complete performance in the domains of 1) hypothesis-directed data gathering, 2) problem representation, 3) prioritized differential diagnosis, 4) addressing high-priority diagnosis, and 5) metacognition (or the awareness of one's thinking process and factors that affect the process) (Thammasitboon et al. 2018). Educating faculty about the tool before use is recommended. Unlike CSR, ART can be used on the fly in clinical situations or in conjunction with CSR.

Faculty assessments are "global assessments that include a rating scale and section for written comments" (Holmboe and Iobst 2020, p. 17). The rating scales and questions can provide ratings of learners within several evaluation frameworks. Faculty assessment forms lack strong intra- and interrater reliability. Most of the variability comes from inadequate or nonexistent faculty development and consensus. Increasing the number of evaluations and the number of evaluators helps improve validity. Faculty global assessment forms are convenient, but a lengthy form that is not fit for the purpose can result in low acceptability.

Clinical performance or *record review* involves critical review of the medical record. This can be performed by automated extraction of data from an electronic medical record or by manual review of the medical record by the student or a reviewer. Adequate manual reviews typically require 10–30 minutes. Sufficient reliability for formative assessment purposes requires reviewing 8–10 of the learner's medical records (Holmboe and Iobst 2020). Note that clinical performance or record review differs from CSR in that CSR incorporates the exploration of clinical reasoning with a set of questions. Significant data support the validity and reliability of clinical performance review. A problem with chart review is attributing patient outcomes to a single person (i.e., the student) when a team of providers contributed to the patient's care (Holmboe and Iobst 2020). Pairing clinical performance review with coaching and a pathway for improving performance can improve the acceptability and catalytic effect of this tool.

Simulation is the use of actors or technology to create an artificial environment that resembles, as closely as possible, a real clinical experience. Simulation allows for assessment on the *Shows how* level of Miller's pyramid (Miller 1990). Simulation is well accepted for formative assessment and variably accepted for summative assessment. A strength of simulation is its strong catalytic effect on learning. Simulation is especially helpful in assessing student performance in rare but serious clinical situations, especially "when mastery-based learning principles are incorporated into the simulation design and experience" (Holmboe and Iobst 2020, p. 27). *Standardized patients* and objective structured clinical examinations (OSCEs) are forms of simulation. OSCEs employ a consistent set of standardized patients at separate stations to assess students. Ample evidence supports the content validity and reliability of OSCEs; less evidence suggests correlations with other assessment data or predictions of future performance. A drawback is the amount of time it takes to train the standardized patient. Regardless, OSCEs have become "a staple of education, training, and assessment in undergraduate medical education" (Holmboe and Iobst 2020, p. 30).

Direct observation is considered a work-based assessment strategy. Direct observation refers to watching a learner perform a clinical task in the workplace for the purpose of assessing the learner. Any clinical task can be observed and assessed. Commonly observed clinical tasks include taking a medical history, performing a mental status examination, or obtaining informed consent. Direct observation assesses what a student *Does*, the highest level of performance on Miller's pyramid (Miller 1990). The mini-clinical evaluation exercise and other tools provide structure to and facilitate documentation of direct observation assessments. Obtaining high-reliability assessment with direct observation requires multiple direct-observation assessments, each performed by a different assessor. Lack of a *shared mental model* among faculty and failure to train faculty on the clinical skill being assessed and on good assessment practice all negatively impact the validity of direct-observation assessments. Direct observation is feasible in that it can be done in small windows of time, or "snapshots"; phone apps have been developed to facilitate the process. (One such app is the Direct Observation of Clinical Care app from the Accreditation Council for Graduate Medical Education [ACGME].) If performed well (frequent assessments, well-trained faculty, and safe learning environments), direct observation has high levels of acceptability. Direct observation provides better data than proxies of clinical care such as presentation of cases in conferences or on rounds. Direct observation provides the foundation of effective feedback and coaching.

Multisource feedback (360-degree feedback) usually involves assessment of the student with the help of a tool (e.g., form, rating scale, questionnaire) by multiple people who have worked with the student, including peers. The strength of 360 feedback is that it provides multiple perspectives on difficult-to-assess competencies such as teamwork, communication, and professionalism. Validity data suggest that multisource feedback can predict future patient complaints and malpractice suits. It is relatively feasible and accepted by teachers and students. Discussing critical multisource feedback results (results with which a student disagrees) with a mentor can facilitate meaningful catalytic effect. ACGME provides a tool called the Teamwork Effectiveness Assessment Module (TEAM).

Patient experience surveys refer to questionnaires that assess patient experience with the care provided during their hospitalizations and outpatient visits. Surveys ask patients to rate prompts such as "I was treated respectfully" and "My questions were answered" on a scale with anchors such as "always" and "never." Reliability requires surveying a lot of patients, and attribution issues can undermine validity, even when using a standardized form such as one of the surveys from the Consumer Assessment of Healthcare Providers and Systems (CAHPS). Even so, patient surveys are necessary, especially in the assessment of interpersonal and communications skills. The relevance of the information provided by patient experience surveys outweighs student acceptability concerns. As for feasibility, a hospital's quality improvement office may have resources. Patient responses to open-ended questions, such as "What did you like or not like about today's appointment?", can also motivate clinical improvement.

Making reliable summative decisions (e.g., whether the medical student has met the required competencies) requires the use of several assessment tools. These tools necessitate several organizational and management issues (e.g., saving and presenting a large number of assessment results in a manner that facilitates 1) the generation of reliable and meaningful feedback and 2) summative decision-making). Educational academicians refer to a group of assessments, their administration, and the management of the data produced as *assessment systems.*

Giving Feedback

The consistent delivery of timely and effective feedback is an essential facet of any successful clerkship program. When administered correctly, feedback can promote medical student learning, encourage attainment of educational benchmarks, and offer trainees invaluable insight into their own areas of strength and weakness (Hewson and

Little 1998). Many physician educators struggle to formulate and deliver feedback that produces the desired effects, and many find the prospect of structured feedback to be uncomfortable or anxiety-inducing. Likewise, surveys of medical students have found that trainees often find their instructors' attempts at providing feedback unhelpful for various reasons (e.g., the feedback is not specific enough, is not appropriate for their level of training, is not based on established goals or competencies, or is perceived as a negative evaluation of the student's abilities rather than an attempt to help them improve) (Brown and Cooke 2009).

This disconnect can lead to dissatisfaction on both sides and hinder the student's growth and improvement. The purpose of this section is to discuss feedback, examine its importance to the psychiatry clerkship, and explore techniques and best practices that promote effective feedback.

What Is Feedback?

For the purpose of this chapter, *feedback* is defined as any information shared with a trainee that concerns their performance and is intended to help them improve. Feedback can take many forms depending on its timing, setting, provider, and intent. Given the potential scope of this topic, it can be helpful to consider medical student clerkship feedback as being divisible into three types (appreciation, coaching, and evaluation), two lengths (brief and extensive), and two styles (informal and formal).

Appreciation

In this context, *appreciation* (also called praise, encouragement, and affirmation) refers to feedback that is generally positive in nature and highlights a student's strengths or acknowledges their efforts. Appreciation is crucial to building rapport with students and reinforcing good habits (Amonoo et al. 2021). Most students enjoy receiving appreciation, and many instructors enjoy giving it. However, studies have shown that praise alone is not effective at improving medical student performance on skills-based assessments (Boehler et al. 2006).

Coaching

Coaching is feedback that consists of specific instructions or suggestions on how to improve a student's performance at a given task. This type of feedback is broad and can range from gentle suggestions on improving study habits after a difficult exam to more stern, in-the-moment correction of a student's unsafe habits observed during patient interactions on the unit. In contrast to appreciation, coaching carries a greater risk of being poorly received by learners, and effective coaching requires greater consideration of its timing, tone, and intent. Coaching-style feedback alone has been shown to be superior to appreciation alone at improving medical student performance, at the expense of student satisfaction (Boehler et al. 2006).

Evaluation

Evaluation is ostensibly the most objective of the three types of feedback in that it directly compares a student's performance to that of their peers or to established expectations. As discussed earlier in this chapter, the setting of clearly defined goals and expectations for students is crucial to the success of any clerkship program, and a major goal of all feedback on the rotation should be to bring students closer to meeting those expectations. Whereas coaching is inherently formative (delivered with the intent of improving performance ahead of a final assessment), evaluation-based feedback is most commonly and effectively used summatively (at the end of an experience to grade a student's performance and explain that mark). Evaluative feedback can also be used during an experience in combination with coaching or appreciation, but drawing direct comparison to peers or standards, rather than the student's own progress, carries the risk of discouraging the student and deemphasizing any other feedback it is paired with (Amonoo et al. 2021).

Brief Versus Extensive Feedback

Again, to be effective, feedback to medical students must be appropriately timed, specific, appropriate for training level, and based on clearly defined expectations. The question, then, becomes, "How do we ensure that students are receiving effective feedback during their psychiatry clerkships, and in appropriate amounts?" A common strategy in clerkships is to encourage a mixture of *brief* feedback and *extensive* feedback.

Brief (or *informal*) *feedback* is relatively short in length (a fair rule of thumb is less than 5 minutes) (Amonoo et al. 2021). Brief feedback is most effective when offered in-the-moment or immediately after a teachable moment, and this type of feedback can occur in any setting.

Its flexible and often impromptu nature means that the majority of brief feedback on the psychiatry clerkship is given verbally and is informal (i.e., unplanned and unrehearsed).

When a larger amount of time, typically 5–20 minutes, is specifically set aside to offer feedback to learners, this constitutes *extensive* (or *formal*) feedback. Examples of extensive feedback include in-depth discussion with a student after a challenging case or patient encounter, planned debriefing sessions after a structured learning activity such as a standardized interview, and scheduled mid- or end-of-rotation feedback meetings. While brief feedback can be used at any time and in a variety of settings, extensive feedback often requires additional consideration of the audience, timing, and location. For example, when extensive feedback is necessary to address a potentially sensitive or embarrassing issue such as a medical error, it is generally best to deliver it in a private setting (Branch and Paranjape 2002).

Giving Effective Feedback

Whenever feedback is given during a clerkship experience, a number of common best practices ensure that the message conveyed is accurate and effective. We recommend that the following techniques be used, regardless of the type of feedback being given.

First, it is crucial to *create a supportive and safe environment,* as students may feel vulnerable or embarrassed when receiving feedback. This type of culture must be promoted through consistent effort on the part of the clerkship director and supervisors—even a single negative interaction or harsh outcome can cause students to feel judged or attacked when receiving feedback in the future. Next, it is often helpful to *elicit learner thoughts and feelings* before delivering feedback. By simply asking, "How do you think that went?" or "What could have been done differently there?", you are giving your student an opportunity to evaluate their own performance and explain their internal process, which can be valuable for guiding your own feedback.

The next two recommendations are closely related: *focus on behaviors* and *be specific*. When offering feedback to a learner during or after a clerkship experience, it can be tempting to critique general aspects of their personality or demeanor (e.g., "You didn't seem interested," "I don't feel like you worked well with the team"). That type of feedback can be difficult for a student to act on and improve. Instead, we recommend identifying specific actions or behaviors the student displayed that led to your evaluation (e.g. "You came across as disinterested when

I saw you on your phone during rounds," "It concerned me when you declined to go with your classmate to see their difficult patient"). This specific and behavior-based feedback identifies clear areas for improvement on future experiences. Finally, after identifying specific behaviors that suggest an area for growth, the instructor should *offer specific advice and solutions*. This can be as simple as providing suggestions for further reading or encouraging students to practice an interaction or procedure to gain confidence; this is also an opportunity to recruit the student into their own improvement strategy by asking, "What can you do to improve on this in the future?"

Conclusions

The prospect of evaluating and giving feedback to medical students during and after their clerkship experience can be daunting for even the most clinically skilled and academically minded physician. It can be tempting to offer only appreciation and avoid use of the much-dreaded but more reliably constructive coaching-type feedback, that will not help students improve their performance on future assessments. By establishing clearly defined standards and expectations, using appropriate assessment and evaluation measures, and consistently delivering appropriately timed, specific, and effective feedback, clerkship directors can efficiently balance student (and instructor) expectations and anxieties surrounding feedback. This balance serves the ultimate goal of the psychiatry clerkship experience: to produce confident and competent physicians who are well acquainted with psychiatric conditions and concepts and who are able to effectively address the mental health needs of their patients.

Key Points

- Assessments performed during educational programs, like clinical rotations, can probe student progress toward achieving educational objectives and provide core information for the construction of meaningful feedback (i.e., formative assessments). Assessments performed at the end of an educational program can provide data to make determinations regarding student achievement of educational objectives and readiness to progress (i.e., summative evaluations).

- The principles of competency-based medical education necessitate assessment of student performance in the clinical workplace.
- Multiple assessment tools are available to probe various domains of medical competence at various levels on Miller's framework. The meaningful demonstration of competence will require the use of multiple assessment methods administered multiple times during the educational program. The optimal group of assessments will vary across medical schools and educational sites.
- Feedback is performance-related information shared with a trainee with the intention of helping them improve.
- Maintaining an environment in which students feel safe and supported increases the educational impact of feedback.

References

Amonoo HL, Longley RM, Robinson DM: Giving feedback. Psychiatr Clin North Am 44(2):237–247, 2021 34049646

assessment. Merriam-Webster.com, 2025. Available at: https://www.merriam-webster.com/dictionary/assessment. Accessed June 3, 2025.

Boehler ML, Rogers DA, Schwind CJ, et al: An investigation of medical student reactions to feedback: a randomised controlled trial. Med Educ 40(8):746–749, 2006 16869919

Branch WT Jr, Paranjape A: Feedback and reflection: teaching methods for clinical settings. Acad Med 77(12 Pt 1):1185–1188, 2002 12480619

Brown N, Cooke L: Giving effective feedback to psychiatric trainees. Adv Psychiatr Treat 15:123–128, 2009

Cheung WJ, Patey AM, Frank JR, et al: Barriers and enablers to direct observation of trainees' clinical performance: a qualitative study using the theoretical domains framework. Acad Med 94(1):101–114, 2019 30095454

Cooke M, Irby DM, O'Brien DC: Educating Physicians: A Call for Reform of Medical School and Residency, in The Preparation for the Professions Series. San Francisco, CA, Jossey-Bass, 2010

Dreyfus SE: The five-stage model of adult skill acquisition. Bull Sci Technol Soc 24(3):177–181, 2004

Frank JR, Snell LS, Cate OT, et al: Competency-based medical education: theory to practice. Med Teach 32(8):638–645, 2010 20662574

Harden RM, Crosby JR, Davis MH, Friedman M: AMEE Guide No. 14: Outcome-based education: Part 5. From competency to meta-competency: a model for the specification of learning outcomes. Med Teach 21(6):546–552, 1999 21281173

Hewson MG, Little ML: Giving feedback in medical education: verification of recommended techniques. J Gen Intern Med 13(2):111–116, 1998 9502371

Holmboe E, Iobst W: Assessment Guidebook. Accreditation Council for Graduate Medical Education, 2020. Available from: https://www.acgme.org/globalassets/pdfs/milestones/guidebooks/assessmentguidebook.pdf. Accessed June 28, 2024.

Liaison Committee on Medical Education: Functions and Structure of a Medical School. LCME, 2023. Available at: https://lcme.org/wp-content/uploads/2025/03/2024-25-Functions-and-Structure_2025-03-07.docx. Accessed June 28, 2024.

Massie J, Ali JM: Workplace-based assessment: a review of user perceptions and strategies to address the identified shortcomings. Adv Health Sci Educ 21:455–473, 2016

Miller GE: The assessment of clinical skills/competence/performance. Acad Med 65(9)(Suppl):S63–S67, 1990 2400509

Norcini J, Anderson B, Bollela V, et al: Criteria for good assessment: consensus statement and recommendations from the Ottawa 2010 Conference. Med Teach 33(3):206–214, 2011 21345060

Norcini J, Anderson MB, Bollela V, et al: 2018 Consensus framework for good assessment. Med Teach 40(11):1102–1109, 2018 30299187

Thammasitboon S, Rencic JJ, Trowbridge RL, et al: The Assessment of Reasoning Tool (ART): structuring the conversation between teachers and learners. Diagnosis (Berl) 5(4):197–203, 2018 30407911

Young JQ, Frank JR, Holmboe ES: Advancing workplace-based assessment in psychiatric education: key design and implementation issues. Psychiatr Clin North Am 44(2):317–332, 2021 34049652

Part III

Teaching Techniques

11

Teaching the Psychiatric Interview to Medical Students

Anuron Mandal, M.D.

The psychiatric interview is the cornerstone of clinical psychiatric practice and an essential skill for medical students to master. It involves a series of structured yet flexible interactions aiming at the development of rapport; the establishment of a comfortable, respectful, and empathetic environment; the gathering of history data; and the proper characterization of the patient's current complaints, personal and family history, medical history, and social aspects (Atkins 2025). Despite the importance of attempting to obtain collateral data from third-party sources whenever possible, the information obtained during the direct interview of the patient remains essential for properly characterizing the patient's history. Moreover, observations made during the psychiatric interview are later used in the description of the patient's mental status examination (MSE) and the preparation of their biopsychosocial formulation, an integrated summary of the biological, psychological, and social factors impacting a patient's mental health and well-being (McClain et al. 2004).

In this chapter, we focus on the priorities and challenges associated with teaching the psychiatric interview to medical students. Even though students should ideally become proficient in how to establish a therapeutic relationship, gather relevant clinical information, make an accurate diagnosis, and develop an appropriate treatment plan, the majority of undergraduate medical students will later pursue specialties other than psychiatry. Therefore, teaching of the psychiatric interview should focus on the best approaches to establish rapport with the patient, obtain essential information, and make preliminary recommendations for purposes of diagnosis and management.

Implementing Effective Teaching Strategies

Effective teaching strategies ensure that medical students not only learn the technical aspects of conducting psychiatric interviews but also develop the soft skills necessary for empathetic and effective patient interactions. Incorporating a diverse range of teaching methods caters to different learning preferences and keeps the educational process engaging and dynamic. Here are some suggested strategies:

1. Interactive lectures: Use lectures to provide foundational knowledge but make them interactive by incorporating questions, live polls, and relevant case discussions. This approach encourages active participation and helps students retain information (Abdel Meguid and Collins 2017).
2. Case-based learning: Case studies are an excellent way for students to apply theoretical knowledge to real-world scenarios (Kalinowski et al. 2020). Supervisors can guide discussion and provide questions for patients to answer using case information.
3. Simulated patient interviews: In addition to direct observation, simulated patient interactions (e.g., standardized patients) allow students to practice interviewing skills in a controlled environment (Siemerkus et al. 2023). Feedback from these sessions is crucial for improving technique and building confidence. Reviewing recordings of these interactions can allow students to identify specific improvement points. Use trained actors to simulate psychiatric interviews, or have residents or faculty members play the role of patients (Hierlihy and Latus 2025). This method still offers realistic scenarios and a controlled environment for

learning. The role of simulation in the teaching of psychiatry to undergraduate medical students is discussed in Chapter 17.

4. Peer learning: Encourage students to work in pairs or small groups to discuss cases, practice interviewing each other, and provide feedback. This peer-to-peer interaction promotes a deeper understanding and appreciation of different perspectives to enhance learning and contribute to the development of clinical skills (Alzaabi et al. 2021).
5. Technology-enhanced learning: Leverage technology such as virtual reality (VR) simulations or online platforms that offer interactive modules and virtual patients (Haowen et al. 2021). These tools can provide immersive experiences that are difficult to replicate in a classroom setting. The use of technology in the teaching of psychiatry is approached in Chapter 16.

Interactions With Real Patients and Teaching the Psychiatric Interview

The didactic approaches outlined in the previous section are of great benefit in providing students with the background and preliminary skills for performing an appropriate psychiatric interview. It is our opinion that experience with actual patients, however—through direct observation of real-life clinical encounters or through the performance of interviews under the supervision and guidance of an instructor or senior resident—is essential for students learning the psychiatric interview. Observing a psychiatric interview as it unfolds or performing a psychiatric interview under supervision provides students with a real-time educational experience that textbooks or lectures cannot replicate. Effective interactions with patients require the mastering of specific interviewing techniques (Gerken et al. 2023; Goto and Takemura 2016). To optimize the educational benefits of a real-world clinical encounter involving students, we suggest a structured approach:

1. Preparation: Set clear educational goals and highlight key aspects of the psychiatric interview to focus on. Provide students with observation guides or checklists that outline the critical components of the psychiatric interview to monitor during the session.

2. Execution: Conduct sessions in a controlled setting where students can witness interviews or perform them without disrupting the clinical flow. Ensure that patient consent and confidentiality are strictly maintained.
3. Debriefing: Facilitate a group discussion to dissect the interview afterward. Explore the techniques and strategies used by the clinician to establish rapport, as well as how sensitive topics were managed. Encourage students to reflect on their observations, focusing on what they learned and how they can apply these insights in their own future practice. After interview sessions, educators can provide immediate feedback and lead discussions, emphasizing key moments and decisions made during the interview. This reinforces learning and addresses any misunderstandings.

Direct Observations

These hands-on experiences allow students to observe real interactions between experienced clinicians and patients, gaining invaluable insight into the nuances of psychiatric assessments. Direct observation and clinical experience bridge the gap between theoretical knowledge and clinical practice. Students observe firsthand how skilled clinicians navigate the complexities of psychiatric interviews, including managing difficult patient interactions and recognizing subtle diagnostic cues. Direct observation allows students to see the professional demeanor, empathy, and communication skills required in psychiatric practice, serving as a model for their future clinical interactions.

Student–Patient Interactions in the Teaching of the Psychiatric Interview

The opportunity of interviewing real-life patients in a clinical setting is of great value for the teaching of the psychiatric interview. Although students are often given the opportunity to ask questions and interact with patients while observing clinical assessments performed by residents or faculty members, it is advisable that, whenever possible, students are given the opportunity to conduct at least one complete interview with a patient, under the supervision of a faculty or senior resident. The instructor should be able to provide feedback about the student's performance once the interview is complete, ask the patient follow-up questions for the purpose of clarification, and occasionally, make interventions over the course of the interview, in case the interview is not progressing properly or safety concerns arise.

Patients to be interviewed by medical students should be selected based on their willingness to do so and their ability to properly engage in the interview. Although students can undoubtedly learn valuable lessons from the experience of interviewing "difficult," manic, hostile, or severely psychotic patients, those are usually not good candidates for students to practice their interviewing skills, as such interactions are often challenging and may become frustrating for inexperienced interviewers. Similarly, as a general rule, it is not advisable that students interview patients who are acutely aggressive or sexually inappropriate. For the same reason, students should always conduct their interviews in an environment that provides physical safety and an easy escape route, especially in the inpatient setting.

From a practical standpoint, students performing a psychiatric interview should be mindful about the following:

- Interview styles: Students are often eager to obtain as much clinical information as possible, sometimes relying on mnemonics and checklists (Caplan and Stern 2008), which can make the interview too inquisitive and have a negative impact on its flow. We encourage students to cultivate a conversational style in the interviews, using open-ended questions (Scardovi et al. 2003) and demonstrating genuine interest in the patient's answers, without being too concerned about time constraints. Reflective and validation statements are valuable approaches for purposes of establishing rapport and should be mastered by students. Moreover, although developing full proficiency in motivational interview is beyond the scope of the psychiatric clerkship, students may benefit from becoming familiar with certain motivational techniques (e.g., the use of affirmations and the use of specific questions aiming at the development of discrepancy) and successfully achieving beginning levels of proficiency (Kaltman and Tankersley 2020). Those techniques may be useful in a variety of clinical situations aiming at eliciting habit change, notably beyond the realm of addictions or even psychiatry.
- Simultaneous assessment of different elements: In somatic medicine, history-taking and the physical examination take place as two separate steps within a clinical encounter; in contrast, the psychiatric interview allows the clinician to concomitantly obtain history data and gather observations to be used later in

the description of the MSE. That process demands some training and familiarity with the different components of the MSE. Students should be instructed to pay attention to nonverbal cues displayed by the patient, such as hygiene and grooming, facial expression and changes when certain topics are discussed, the presence of involuntary movements and other psychomotor abnormalities, and indirect signs of psychosis (self-talking, perplexity, internal preoccupation). Specific questions and other strategies aiming at characterizing the patient's formal cognitive status can be used, but students should also learn how to make inferences about a patient's orientation and memory based on the patient report and its chronology.

- Challenging questions from patients: Students should be instructed about the limits of self-disclosure and about how to deal with questions they do not feel comfortable answering or are not in a position to answer (including questions about the treatment plan, fitness for discharge, and countertransferential feelings that might emerge during the interview). Patients experiencing delusions often ask the interviewers whether they believe in the veracity of their reports; answering that question while still preserving a good therapeutic relationship with the patient can be difficult, even for seasoned clinicians.
- Points of caution: Students should always monitor their countertransferential feelings over the course of the interview. We usually instruct our students in advance with regard to any safety concerns or uncomfortable feelings that might emerge during the interview and tell them to feel comfortable to stop the assessment prematurely if the situation becomes unmanageable. Similarly, students should be prepared in advance about the possibility of patients refusing to be interviewed by them or requesting to interrupt the interview, and about the transferential factors that usually play a role in such situations. This preparation will help students not take such outcomes as a personal affront or an indicator of poor interviewing skills.

Teaching the Mental Status Examination

The MSE is a critical tool for psychiatric assessment, providing a snapshot of a patient's psychological functioning at a specific moment in time. Educators must emphasize the importance of this examination and equip students with the skills to perform it effectively. Some of the approaches to teach the MSE include specific lectures, supplemented with readings from established psychiatric texts, video demonstrations showing real-life scenarios of patient encounters with subsequent exercises on the description of the MSE, and discussions on specific MSE items during the debriefing after direct observation of interviews.

Of note, there is considerable variation in the way the MSE is structured and in the terminology used to characterize its abnormalities (Sanches 2025). A comprehensive discussion of these variations is beyond the scope of this chapter, but we suggest emphasizing the following components when teaching the MSE to medical students:

- Appearance and behavior: Students should be instructed to observe and note physical appearance, attire, posture, and motor behavior, which can provide insight into the patient's psychological state.
- Mood and affect: Guide students on how to assess mood (the patient's subjective experience) and affect (the observable expression of emotion), noting any discrepancies that might be clinically significant.
- Thought process: Train students in the characterization of the rate, continuity, logic, and coherence of speech, for the identification of potential thought disorders.
- Thought content: Students should report specific contents conveyed by the patient, including delusions, depressive thoughts, obsessive thoughts, and suicidal thoughts, among others.
- Sensoperception: Instruct students in the identification of hallucinations and behaviors that indicate ongoing perceptual disturbances during the interview.
- Cognition: Include assessments of orientation, attention, memory, and higher cognitive functions.
- Judgment and insight: Insight is the patient's awareness and acknowledgment of the presence of a mental disorder, and judgment is their ability to reach appropriate conclusions in real or hypothetical situations. The two are often assessed together.

With regard to terminology, it is important to ensure that students are familiar with specific terms used in the description of the MSE. Nevertheless, for purposes of writing notes, we often advise our students to describe the finding or abnormality in question when not sure about the correct psychopathological term.

Teaching the Biopsychosocial Formulation

The biopsychosocial formulation is a comprehensive approach that considers biological, psychological, and social factors influencing a patient's mental health (McClain et al. 2004). Teaching this formulation to medical students is vital for developing a holistic understanding of patient care.

The first step in the teaching of the biopsychosocial formulation should be introducing to students the concept of the biopsychosocial model. Explain how this approach integrates multiple dimensions of a patient's life and health, moving beyond the traditional medical model that focuses solely on biological factors. Emphasize the importance of understanding how psychological aspects (such as emotions, thoughts, and behaviors) and social contexts (such as culture, family dynamics, and socioeconomic status) influence the patient's health and treatment outcomes.

Next, teach students how to gather comprehensive histories that cover all aspects of the biopsychosocial model. Incorporating role-playing exercises into the curriculum can be particularly useful to help students practice biopsychosocial formulations. Create scenarios in which students must assess simulated patients based on detailed backgrounds provided to them. After the role-play, have them present their biopsychosocial formulations to the class for feedback and discussion. Encourage critical thinking by presenting complex case scenarios in which students need to develop a biopsychosocial formulation that addresses conflicting or ambiguous information. Use group discussions to facilitate problem-solving, allowing students to debate and reason through different perspectives to find the most comprehensive understanding of the case.

During patient interviews, guide students on how to ask open-ended questions that explore not just physical symptoms but also psychological experiences and social environments. For instance, questions might explore family mental health history, personal relationships, job stress, and community involvement, all of which provide insight into the patient's biopsychosocial health. Provide detailed feedback on students' biopsychosocial formulations, focusing on their ability to integrate diverse information into a coherent profile of the patient. Encourage students to revise their formulations based on feedback, which helps them learn the iterative nature of clinical thinking and improves their diagnostic and treatment-planning skills.

Teaching the biopsychosocial formulation requires an integrated approach that highlights the interconnectedness of biological, psychological, and social factors. By using these teaching strategies, educators can prepare medical students to consider all aspects of a patient's life and health in their future clinical practice, leading to more comprehensive and effective patient care.

Specific Topics in the Teaching of the Psychiatric Interview

Risk Assessment

Risk assessment, an integral part of the psychiatric interview, is essential to determine the immediate safety needs of the patient and others (Shea 2017). Introduce to students the concept of risk, emphasizing that some risk factors for suicide and aggression are to be acknowledged, and others are potentially modifiable. To perform a risk assessment, students should be proficient in the following:

- Red flags: Educate students on recognizing key indicators of risk such as history of self-harm or violent behavior; suicidal thoughts, plans, means, or intentions; and signs of potential violence.
- Environmental and social considerations: Discuss the importance of considering the patient's current support system, living conditions, and recent stressors or life changes.
- Safety planning: Instruct students on how to develop effective safety plans that include patient and family education, emergency contacts, limiting access to means, and the importance of follow-up care arrangements.

In addition to discussions on risk assessment during encounters with real patients, different teaching strategies can be used to introduce students to the process of risk assessment in psychiatry. For example, case studies illustrate various risky scenarios and the most appropriate responses to them. Facilitate discussions on hypothetical scenarios where students must decide how to handle different levels of risk, including identifying potential for suicide and violence; this exercise helps students develop critical thinking and decision-making skills.

The Differential Diagnosis Between Psychiatric and Somatic Conditions

Somatic conditions often present with psychiatric symptoms (Frumin et al. 1998; Marsh 1997). Even though most students will not pursue psychiatry as a medical specialty, developing familiarity with the differential diagnosis between primary psychiatric disorders and somatic conditions that present with psychiatric symptoms is an important aspect of their undergraduate psychiatric training. Students should be educated about certain clinical and epidemiological features that raise suspicion about a possible medical etiology during a psychiatric interview:

- Late onset of symptoms in a patient without prior psychiatric history. Instruct your students about the usual age of onset of most common psychiatric conditions and encourage them to consider the differential with a neurological or medical condition among patients who show marked deviation from that age. Encourage the use of cognitive screening tools, such as the Mini-Mental State Examination and the Montreal Cognitive Assessment (Folstein et al. 1975; Ismail et al. 2010; Nasreddine et al. 2005) when a neurocognitive disorder is suspected.
- Sudden onset of symptoms in patients with no previous psychiatric history and fluctuation in symptomatology and mental status. Although many psychiatric conditions can present with sudden onset, acute onset of symptoms with waxing and waning course may be an indication of delirium.
- Comorbid medical conditions or the presence of physical symptoms temporarily associated with the onset of psychiatric symptoms. Help students develop critical thinking/skepticism regarding the possible role of certain medical conditions as an etiology for psychiatric complaints, such as hypothyroidism, diabetes, cerebrovascular disease, seizures, and others. Educate students about the importance of performing a full review of systems while performing a psychiatric assessment, including questions about the use of medications for medical issues, and encourage them to carry out a focused physical examination when appropriate.
- Specific psychiatric symptoms. Students should be aware of certain red-flag symptoms that raise concerns about a possible medical etiology, such as visual hallucinations (especially in the

absence of associated delusions) and grossly impaired level of consciousness with inattention and severe disorientation. Teach your students how to perform easy, quick tests to screen for possible impairment in level of consciousness, such as serial subtractions or listing the months of the year forward and backward.

Furthermore, if a somatic etiology is suspected, students should be familiar with the best next steps to confirm or rule out that possibility, including laboratory tests, brain imaging tests, and obtaining a clinical or neurological assessment. In certain settings or urgent situations, that may include referring the patient to the emergency department or requesting support from emergency medical services.

Challenges and Solutions in Teaching the Psychiatric Interview

Teaching the psychiatric interview presents unique challenges, related to both the complexity of the skills required and the potentially sensitive nature of clinical situations. The following challenges should be considered in addition to the specific issues discussed earlier in this chapter.

- Diverse learning preferences: Students usually have different learning preferences and learning paces, which can complicate the teaching of complex skills such as psychiatric interviewing. Ensure that students' initial real-patient interviews are closely supervised by experienced clinicians who can provide immediate feedback and intervention if necessary. Implement a robust feedback system in which students can receive constructive criticism on their interviewing techniques and overall approach. Encourage a culture of peer review in which students can critique each other's approach in a supportive environment, promoting mutual learning and improvement.
- Balancing theory and practice: Finding the right balance between theoretical knowledge and practical experience can be challenging, as both are essential for mastering psychiatric interviewing. Develop the habit of offering your students reading materials; if time allows, encourage group discussions of these materials.
- Dealing with sensitive topics: Students may feel uncomfortable or unprepared when they first deal with sensitive topics such

as suicide, abuse, or severe mental illness during interviews. Workshops or seminars focusing specifically on how to handle sensitive topics during psychiatric interviews can be of benefit. Additionally, offer regular debriefing sessions after patient interviews to help students process their experiences, reinforce learning, and address any emotional effects.

Providing Effective Feedback on Interview Techniques to Medical Students

As noted at different points during this chapter, feedback is an essential component of educational training, particularly in the context of teaching psychiatric interviewing skills. It helps students refine their techniques, develop professionalism, and enhance their interpersonal skills. For a deeper discussion on providing feedback to medical students, please see Chapter 10, "Assessment and Feedback to Medical Students During Psychiatry Rotations."

Conclusions

Teaching the psychiatric interview to medical students may be particularly challenging, given the multitude of aspects involved. Educators should strive to adopt a structured approach while instructing medical students in performing the psychiatric interview, emphasizing the importance of the interview while maintaining a respectful environment for patients and trainees.

Key Points

- The psychiatric interview is the cornerstone of clinical psychiatric practice, and conducting the psychiatric interview is an essential skill for medical students to master.
- Direct observation and feedback are essential tools while teaching the psychiatric interview.
- Different teaching techniques can be used to teach the psychiatric interview to medical students.

References

Abdel Meguid E, Collins M: Students' perceptions of lecturing approaches: traditional versus interactive teaching. Adv Med Educ Pract 8:229–241, 2017 28360541

Alzaabi S, Nasaif M, Khamis AH, et al: Medical students' perception and perceived value of peer learning in undergraduate clinical skill development and assessment: mixed methods study. JMIR Med Educ 7(3):e25875, 2021 34021539

Atkins D: The Psychiatric Interview, in Fundamentals of Clinical Psychiatry: A Practical Handbook, edited by Sanches M, Soares JC. Cambridge, UK, Cambridge University Press, 2025

Caplan JP, Stern TA: Mnemonics in a mnutshell: 32 aids to psychiatric diagnosis; clever, irreverent, or amusing, a mnemonic you remember is a lifelong learning tool. Curr Psychiatr 7(10):27, 2008

Folstein MF, Folstein SE, McHugh PR: "Mini-Mental State": a practical method for grading the cognitive state of patients for the clinician. J Psychiatr Res 12(3):189–198, 1975 1202204

Frumin M, Chisholm T, Dickey CC, Daffner KR: Psychiatric and behavioral problems. Neurol Clin 16(2):521–544, 1998 9537973

Gerken AT, Beckmann DL, Stoklosa JB: Interviewing a patient experiencing psychosis. Curr Psychiatr 22(11):48–49, 2023

Goto M, Takemura YC: Which medical interview skills are associated with patients' verbal indications of undisclosed feelings of anxiety and depressive feelings? Asia Pac Fam Med 15(1):2, 2016 26924940

Haowen J, Vimalesvaran S, Myint Kyaw B, Tudor Car L: Virtual reality in medical students' education: a scoping review protocol. BMJ Open 11(5):e046986, 2021 34039577

Hierlihy T, Latus A: An approach to teaching the psychiatric interview. BMC Med Educ 25(1):110, 2025 39849526

Ismail Z, Rajji TK, Shulman KI: Brief cognitive screening instruments: an update. Int J Geriatr Psychiatry 25(2):111–120, 2010 19582756

Kalinowski A, Raj KS, Bandstra BS: Teaching practice-based learning on inpatient psychiatric services. Acad Psychiatry 44(1):86–89, 2020 31642050

Kaltman S, Tankersley A: Teaching motivational interviewing to medical students: a systematic review. Acad Med 95(3):458–469, 2020 31577585

Marsh CM: Psychiatric presentations of medical illness. Psychiatr Clin North Am 20(1):181–204, 1997 9139290

McClain T, O'Sullivan PS, Clardy JA: Biopsychosocial formulation: recognizing educational shortcomings. Acad Psychiatry 28(2):88–94, 2004 15298859

Nasreddine ZS, Phillips NA, Bédirian V, et al: The Montreal Cognitive Assessment, MoCA: a brief screening tool for mild cognitive impairment. J Am Geriatr Soc 53(4):695–699, 2005 15817019

Sanches M: Psychopathology and the Mental Status Examination, in Fundamentals of Clinical Psychiatry: A Practical Handbook. Edited by Sanches M, Soares JC. Cambridge, UK, Cambridge University Press, 2025

Scardovi A, Rucci P, Gask L, et al: Improving psychiatric interview skills of established GPs: evaluation of a group training course in Italy. Fam Pract 20(4):363–369, 2003 12876103

Shea SC: Psychiatric Interviewing: The Art of Understanding, 3rd Edition. New York, Elsevier, 2017

Siemerkus J, Petrescu A-S, Köchli L, et al: Using standardized patients for undergraduate clinical skills training in an introductory course to psychiatry. BMC Med Educ 23(1):159, 2023 36922802

12

Clinical Pearls in Psychiatry: What All Students Should Know

Michael McClam, M.D.

Clinical pearls are "small bits of freestanding clinically relevant information based on experience or observation" (Lorin et al. 2008). It is difficult to summarize psychiatry in terms of clinical pearls. As a senior clinician, I may have more experience than most, but I still have a lot to learn about the field. The complexity of psychiatric diagnosis, particularly as it manifests in the clinical setting, makes it difficult to distill it into a "one-size-fits-all" clinical pearl that applies to every circumstance.

The beginning student, however, needs a jumping-off point to help guide their understanding and learning of psychiatry. Clinical pearls may not be applicable to every case, but they are good enough to apply to many cases, and they may give students a sense of direction when learning about psychiatry.

Psychiatric conditions are a part of, and manifest in, every aspect of clinical medicine. When someone becomes sick with a medical illness, that person could have a range of responses partly based on the diagnosis and its severity (as relayed by the physician). In addition, how a person responds to illness speaks to how they approach adversity—in other words, a person's life experiences, personality, ability to interact with people, and reaction to difficulties also inform their response to illness. To complicate matters further, preexisting depression, anxiety, or psychosis can affect a patient's perspective on and adaptive responses to illnesses.

The Use of Observation to Help Develop or Confirm Clinical Hypotheses

Consider the power of observation in patient interactions that may help guide your questions to students about an illness or may help direct students to notice nonverbal information that can help make clinical decisions. For example, how does a patient look in general? Do they look the examiner in the eyes or divert away? If they divert their gaze, is there a specific topic or time in the interview that it happened? How about their tone of voice? Are they yelling or can you barely hear them? What about the person's general appearance? Are they neat and clean, with everything in place, or disheveled? Does the tone of their voice or facial expression match the content of the conversation, or does it seem inconsistent? How about the actual content? Are they making sense? Can you follow the associations they are making over the course of the conversation, or do they seem to jump all over the place?

These are some of the prompts you can use to direct learning during the course of an interview, without having to ask the patient. The learner should come to understand that you're noticing nonverbal subtleties to give you more information.

Issues Facing Early-Career Learners When Diagnosing Psychiatric Conditions

At the forefront of a student's tasks is learning how to diagnose psychiatric disorders. Descriptions of illnesses such as depression, anxiety, schizophrenia, and personality disorders are found in the *Diagnostic and Statistical Manual of Mental Disorders* (DSM). DSM was first produced in the 1950s by the American Psychiatric Association to provide a common diagnostic language for practicing clinicians and to gather and classify data about psychiatric diagnoses for research and statistical purposes. Over the decades, DSM has undergone revision as psychiatrists and other mental health clinicians have refined what actually constitutes a psychiatric diagnosis. The most recent revision, the fifth (American Psychiatric Association 2013), is notably more sensitive to cultural factors that influence clinical presentations of psychiatric illness. The fifth edition underwent a text revision (updated without significant changes to diagnostic criteria), referred to as DSM-5-TR (American Psychiatric Association 2022).

DSM is a text created by expert consensus, describing the symptoms (as opposed to laboratory studies, testing, or other diagnostic studies) whose presence indicates a certain mental illness. In other words, all of the major diagnostic entities in DSM are clinical: diagnoses are based primarily on observing signs and symptoms of the patient in real time, deducing symptoms from other clues (including the descriptions of collateral sources close to the patient), and determining whether the symptoms cause significant functional impairment and are not caused by either the intoxication of or withdrawal from a substance or the consequence of a medical illness.

It is important to note that psychiatric diagnoses are diagnoses of exclusion. If someone exhibits symptoms consistent with a psychiatric disorder, it may actually be caused by something else that, when treated, will relieve the symptoms. In other words, in someone showing a change in behavior from baseline, that change could be caused by a medical condition or substance use. For example, if a patient presents with sad mood, decreased energy, fatigue, and difficulty with concentration, they do not necessarily have a diagnosis of major depression. The clinician has to prove that it is not caused by something else.

To reiterate, psychiatric diagnoses are diagnoses of exclusion. Take a look at the DSM diagnostic criteria for major depressive disorder (Table 12.1).

Notice that, embedded in the diagnostic criteria, the language asserting that the depressive episode is "not attributable to the physiological effects of a substance or another medical condition." Some medical diagnoses (e.g., low blood sugar, anemia, viral infection, or vitamin deficiency), medications (e.g., interferons, benzodiazepines), or substances can cause depression. A careful interview, reviewing with the patient all the possible complicating factors, will help rule out those conditions that can confuse the diagnosis.

Table 12.1 Diagnostic criteria for major depressive disorder

A. Five (or more) of the following symptoms have been present during the same 2-week period and represent a change from previous functioning; at least one of the symptoms is either (1) depressed mood or (2) loss of interest or pleasure.

Note: Do not include symptoms that are clearly attributable to another medical condition.

1. Depressed mood most of the day, nearly every day, as indicated by either subjective report (e.g., feels sad, empty, hopeless) or observation made by others (e.g., appears tearful). (**Note:** In children and adolescents, can be irritable mood.)

2. Markedly diminished interest or pleasure in all, or almost all, activities most of the day, nearly every day (as indicated by either subjective account or observation).

3. Significant weight loss when not dieting or weight gain (e.g., a change of more than 5% of body weight in a month), or decrease or increase in appetite nearly every day. (**Note:** In children, consider failure to make expected weight gain.)

4. Insomnia or hypersomnia nearly every day.

5. Psychomotor agitation or retardation nearly every day (observable by others, not merely subjective feelings of restlessness or being slowed down).

6. Fatigue or loss of energy nearly every day.

7. Feelings of worthlessness or excessive or inappropriate guilt (which may be delusional) nearly every day (not merely self-reproach or guilt about being sick).

8. Diminished ability to think or concentrate, or indecisiveness, nearly every day (either by subjective account or as observed by others).

9. Recurrent thoughts of death (not just fear of dying); recurrent suicidal ideation without a specific plan; a specific suicide plan; or a suicide attempt.

B. The symptoms cause clinically significant distress or impairment in social, occupational, or other important areas of functioning.

C. The episode is not attributable to the physiological effects of a substance or another medical condition.

Note: Criteria A–C represent a major depressive episode.

Table 12.1 Diagnostic criteria for major depressive disorder *(continued)*
Note: Responses to a significant loss (e.g., bereavement, financial ruin, losses from a natural disaster, a serious medical illness or disability) may include the feelings of intense sadness, rumination about the loss, insomnia, poor appetite, and weight loss noted in Criterion A, which may resemble a depressive episode. Although such symptoms may be understandable or considered appropriate to the loss, the presence of a major depressive episode in addition to the normal response to a significant loss should also be carefully considered. This decision inevitably requires the exercise of clinical judgment based on the individual's history and the cultural norms for the expression of distress in the context of loss.
D. At least one major depressive episode is not better explained by schizoaffective disorder and is not superimposed on schizophrenia, schizophreniform disorder, delusional disorder, or other specified or unspecified schizophrenia spectrum and other psychotic disorders.
E. There has never been a manic episode or a hypomanic episode.
NOTE: This exclusion does not apply if all of the manic-like or hypomanic-like episodes are substance-induced or are attributable to the physiological effects of another medical condition.

Source. Reprinted from American Psychiatric Association: *Diagnostic and Statistical Manual of Mental Disorders*, 5th Edition, Text Revision. Washington, DC, American Psychiatric Association, 2022, p. 183.

Not all behavioral changes are diagnosed as psychiatric. DSM stipulates that the symptoms a patient describes must "cause clinically significant distress or impairment in social, occupational, or other important areas of functioning." In other words, the symptoms have to get in the way of what a person wants to do or their ability to live the life they want to live.

DSM provides the clinician with a template to use in diagnosing psychiatric disorders, but using it in an effective way can be a challenge. It provides a listing of symptoms, a time course of symptoms, and some conditions to consider (or better yet, exclude) before diagnosing a psychiatric disorder. But how does a clinician actually do that? The interview is key to developing a working diagnosis for a patient.

With all this in mind, below are some clinical pearls to help the learner navigate when interviewing patients, thinking about differential diagnosis, and formulating a psychiatric diagnosis when appropriate.

Clinical Pearls to Help With Psychiatric Diagnosis

Clinical Pearl 1: Look for Other Causes of the Observed Mental Changes

Many conditions, particularly medical diagnoses, can be treated and resolved; others can complicate diagnosis or treatment. For example, a person with anemia can have symptoms that resemble depression, such as fatigue, loss of interest in previously enjoyed activities, or lack of focus. Electrolyte disturbances can alter a person's mental status; when they are corrected, the altered mental status is also corrected. Delirium—altered mental status caused by a medical condition—is corrected only when the medical condition is addressed. Substances of abuse, such as alcohol, stimulants, medications such as sedatives, or some types of blood pressure medications, can simulate psychiatric symptoms that resolve once the substance is cleared from the body. The upshot is, many conditions, substances, or medications can manifest as or mimic behavioral or psychiatric issues. Making sure those likely causes are investigated and resolved is crucial before diagnosing a "pure" psychiatric illness.

Clinical Pearl 2: Patients With a Confirmed Psychiatric Diagnosis Can Have Medical Problems, Too

Patients often use physical symptoms to communicate psychological problems, complicating the task of diagnosis for both junior and senior clinicians. Because of the stigma associated with psychiatric diagnoses, presenting with physical symptoms may be more acceptable or generate more attention. If a person receives a thorough medical workup and no clear medical problems are found, they may be told, "It's all in your head." That kind of statement leads to shame and guilt, further dissuading the patient from seeking treatment. A patient who uses medical issues repeatedly to express psychological problems may be dismissed by medical professionals when in fact they have a somatic issue that needs treatment.

Clinical Pearl 3: Observation Is Just as Helpful in Discerning Psychiatric Diagnoses as the Patient's Words

Does the patient look disheveled? Does the patient make strange movements? Not just what a patient says, but how they say it, is important. Can you follow along with their train of thought? Are they barely speaking in a whisper, or yelling angrily? If there is opportunity, just observing a patient in their surroundings and how they interact with others may provide valuable insight into how they think about themselves and how they use relationships to meet their emotional, social, or psychological needs.

Clinical Pearl 4: Sometimes to Get to the Heart of the Matter, You Need to Talk to Someone Besides the Patient

Sometimes, when a patient provides their history, it can be incoherent, inconsistent, or confusing as to the timeline; sometimes, the patient does not want to speak or is incapacitated. In that case, other people in the patient's life can offer valuable insight into the patient's social environment, behavior, general functioning, or decline in functioning in the period leading up to their presentation. A collateral source, such as a relative or friend, may also be able to tell you how they experience the patient, particularly before the current crisis. You can use that information to think about how their experience compares to your own interaction with the patient.

Clinical Pearl 5: Timing Is Everything

Many diagnoses are differentiated by time. For example, the main thing that separates brief psychotic disorder from schizophreniform illnesses is the time course. In Table 12.2, Table 12.3, and Table 12.4, the symptoms in criterion A are similar, but the time course for schizophrenia (criteria B and C) and schizophreniform disorder (criterion B) differ significantly from that of brief psychotic disorder. Getting as

Table 12.2 Diagnostic criteria for brief psychotic disorder

A. Presence of one (or more) of the following symptoms. At least one of these must be (1), (2), or (3):

1. Delusions.
2. Hallucinations.
3. Disorganized speech (e.g., frequent derailment or incoherence).
4. Grossly disorganized or catatonic behavior.

Note: Do not include a symptom if it is a culturally sanctioned response.

B. Duration of an episode of the disturbance is at least 1 day but less than 1 month, with eventual full return to premorbid level of functioning.

C. The disturbance is not better explained by major depressive or bipolar disorder with psychotic features or another psychotic disorder such as schizophrenia or catatonia, and is not attributable to the physiological effects of a substance (e.g., a drug of abuse, a medication) or another medical condition.

Source. Reprinted from American Psychiatric Association: *Diagnostic and Statistical Manual of Mental Disorders,* 5th Edition, Text Revision. Washington, DC, American Psychiatric Association, 2022, pp. 108–109.

solid a timeline as possible will make a difference in diagnosing a psychiatric disorder.

So, when asking about time, be as specific as possible. How long have the symptoms lasted? A few days? A month? For example, normal sadness may last for only a few days to a week and does not mean that a person has major depression. Grief is normal, but a patient who displays symptoms of acute grief for more than 6 months may have prolonged grief disorder. Adjustment disorders, by definition, last at least 6 months. So timing is key to discerning many psychiatric diagnoses.

Clinical Pearl 6: Small Talk With a Patient Is Not Just Okay, It Is Really Helpful in Your Mental Status Examination

There are standardized instruments you can use to determine overall mental status, including general cognition, working memory, figure

Table 12.3 Diagnostic criteria for schizophrenia

A. Two (or more) of the following, each present for a significant portion of time during a 1-month period (or less if successfully treated). At least one of these must be (1), (2), or (3):

1. Delusions.
2. Hallucinations.
3. Disorganized speech (e.g., frequent derailment or incoherence).
4. Grossly disorganized or catatonic behavior.
5. Negative symptoms (i.e., diminished emotional expression or avolition).

B. For a significant portion of the time since the onset of the disturbance, level of functioning in one or more major areas, such as work, interpersonal relations, or self-care, is markedly below the level achieved prior to the onset (or when the onset is in childhood or adolescence, there is failure to achieve expected level of interpersonal, academic, or occupational functioning).

C. Continuous signs of the disturbance persist for at least 6 months. This 6-month period must include at least 1 month of symptoms (or less if successfully treated) that meet Criterion A (i.e., active-phase symptoms) and may include periods of prodromal or residual symptoms. During these prodromal or residual periods, the signs of the disturbance may be manifested by only negative symptoms or by two or more symptoms listed in Criterion A present in an attenuated form (e.g., odd beliefs, unusual perceptual experiences).

D. Schizoaffective disorder and depressive or bipolar disorder with psychotic features have been ruled out because either 1) no major depressive or manic episodes have occurred concurrently with the active-phase symptoms, or 2) if mood episodes have occurred during active-phase symptoms, they have been present for a minority of the total duration of the active and residual periods of the illness.

E. The disturbance is not attributable to the physiological effects of a substance (e.g., a drug of abuse, a medication) or another medical condition.

F. If there is a history of autism spectrum disorder or a communication disorder of childhood onset, the additional diagnosis of schizophrenia is made only if prominent delusions or hallucinations, in addition to the other required symptoms of schizophrenia, are also present for at least 1 month (or less if successfully treated).

Source. Reprinted from American Psychiatric Association: *Diagnostic and Statistical Manual of Mental Disorders*, 5th Edition, Text Revision. Washington, DC, American Psychiatric Association, 2022, pp. 113–114.

recognition, recall, and rudimentary executive functioning (i.e., whether the person can follow simple directions). Small talk, however, can do many of the same things. At the same time, small talk helps you as a clinician establish rapport or develop some points of connection with a patient. For example, asking where the patient is from may spark a common background or interest in that area. Asking what interests they have (running, reading, playing games, etc.) can demonstrate a patient's ability to recall, their working memory, their ability to keep a train of thought, their general behavior (pleasant? labile? guarded?), and whether they are oriented. Usually, outpatients who keep an appointment at the clinic or office on their own are oriented (i.e., they have

Table 12.4 **Diagnostic criteria for schizophreniform disorder**

A. Two (or more) of the following, each present for a significant portion of time during a 1-month period (or less if successfully treated). At least one of these must be (1), (2), or (3):

1. Delusions.
2. Hallucinations.
3. Disorganized speech (e.g., frequent derailment or incoherence).
4. Grossly disorganized or catatonic behavior.
5. Negative symptoms (i.e., diminished emotional expression or avolition).

B. An episode of the disorder lasts at least 1 month but less than 6 months. When the diagnosis must be made without waiting for recovery, it should be qualified as "provisional."

C. Schizoaffective disorder and depressive or bipolar disorder with psychotic features have been ruled out because either 1) no major depressive or manic episodes have occurred concurrently with the active-phase symptoms, or 2) if mood episodes have occurred during active-phase symptoms, they have been present for a minority of the total duration of the active and residual periods of the illness.

D. The disturbance is not attributable to the physiological effects of a substance (e.g., a drug of abuse, a medication) or another medical condition.

Source. Reprinted from American Psychiatric Association: *Diagnostic and Statistical Manual of Mental Disorders,* 5th Edition, Text Revision. Washington, DC, American Psychiatric Association, 2022, p. 111.

enough situational awareness to know the time and place and enough executive functioning to plan a trip from where they live or work to get to the clinic on time). No such assumptions can be made about patients who are escorted by a caregiver, however. If feasible, a conversation with the caregiver may give you crucial collateral information about the patient's overall functioning outside the clinic. Of course, speaking with the patient directly or using one of the standardized measures mentioned earlier will help.

Clinical Pearl 7: Always Consider Social and Cultural Factors in the Presentation of Distress, Response to Injury, or Psychiatric Illness

Many medical texts—and therefore, the learning perspective—have been written through a Western, Eurocentric, cis-gendered, heterosexual, medium-to-high socioeconomic lens. It should be obvious, but there is a need to state it anyway: Not every patient has that perspective. Patients' unique perspectives affect their perception of illness, whether their distress is viewed as a psychiatric illness, and what interventions would be most helpful in ameliorating their symptoms (or at least providing comfort). For some, their positioning outside the traditional White, binary culture is a stressor in and of itself and affects access to and trust in the medical system. Over the years, so-called culture-bound syndromes were delineated to describe distress displayed by indigenous and other groups as observed by Western psychiatrists. A more careful review revealed that those syndromes were being viewed from a hierarchical perspective—e.g., a "more sophisticated" culture judging other cultures as less sophisticated.

Clinical Pearl 8: Do Not Be Afraid to Talk About Suicide and Self-Harm

The topic of suicide is fraught with anxiety for any clinician of any skill level or experience. Suicide is the second leading cause of death for young adults aged 15–24 and the tenth leading cause of death for adults in the United States. Many individuals who report suicidal thinking have a history of mental illness, but be aware that some do not, and their first presentation to a medical professional may be thoughts of suicide independent of a previously diagnosed mental illness. A common myth is that talking about suicide with a depressed patient may "induce" suicidal thinking. In fact, that does not occur. Many patients suffer in silence; stigma about mental health in general may be a barrier for them to be talk about their suicidal thinking. Talking about it helps break the stigma and allows patients to open up about their experience. Taking a nonjudgmental stance and using active listening will help you in gathering more details about the patient's thoughts, intents, or plans. Moreover, being open about suicide can help with risk assessment and taking action as necessary to keep a patient safe, such as calling for support (911, the suicide hotline 988, or in a hospital setting, senior members of the clinical team such as the resident or attending) or securing hospitalization.

Conclusions

These clinical pearls are but a small starter sample for a beginner's journey into the world of psychiatry. To recap:

1. Look for other causes of the observed changes in mental status (medical conditions, substances).
2. Patients with a confirmed psychiatric diagnosis can have medical problems, too.
3. Observation is just as helpful in discerning psychiatric diagnoses as the patient's words.
4. Sometimes to get to the heart of the matter, you'll need to talk to someone besides the patient.
5. Timing is everything: many diagnoses are separated by time.
6. Small talk with a patient is not just okay, it is really helpful in your mental status examination.
7. Always consider social or cultural factors and how they may affect psychiatric illness.
8. Do not be afraid to talk about suicide and self-harm.

With these pearls in mind, a learner should be prepared to think about interviewing, gathering collateral information, discussing, and diagnosing psychiatric conditions or discerning if other medical interventions should be considered.

Key Points

- Clinical pearls are small, specific pieces of clinically relevant information based on experience or observation
- The formulation of broadly applicable pearls may be particularly challenging, given the complexities of psychiatry and the multiple factors involved in a case assessment, formulation, and management. Nevertheless, for medical students being introduced to the field of psychiatry, clinical pearls offered by clinician-educators may provide a sense of direction.

Suggested Reading

Folstein MF, Folstein SE, McHugh PR: "Mini-Mental State": a practical method for grading the cognitive state of patients for the clinician. J Psychiatr Res 12(3):189–198, 1975 1202204

Jacobs DG, Brewer M, Klein-Benheim M: Suicide Assessment: An Overview and Recommended Protocol, in The Harvard Medical School Guide to Suicide Assessment and Intervention. Edited by Jacobs DG. New York, Jossey-Bass/Wiley, 1999, pp 3–39

Nasreddine ZS, Phillips NA, Bédirian V, et al: Montreal Cognitive Assessment, MoCA: a brief screening tool for mild cognitive impairment. J Am Geriatr Soc 53(4):695–699, 2005

Tseng WS: From peculiar psychiatric disorders through culture-bound syndromes to culture-related specific syndromes. Transcult Psychiatry 43(4):554–576, 2006 17166946

References

American Psychiatric Association: Diagnostic and Statistical Manual of Mental Disorders, 5th Edition. Arlington, VA, American Psychiatric Association, 2013

American Psychiatric Association: Diagnostic and Statistical Manual of Mental Disorders, 5th Edition, Text Revision. Washington, DC, American Psychiatric Association, 2022

Lorin MI, Palazzi DL, Turner TL, Ward MA: What is a clinical pearl and what is its role in medical education? Med Teach 30(9–10):870–874, 2008

13

Ten Psychiatry Reading Materials I Recommend to My Students

Serena M. Weber, M.D.
Neil V. Puri, M.D.

As medical students transition to clinical experiences, they learn how to apply their fundamental medical knowledge to clinical practice. Students also start encountering diseases they previously knew only in didactic settings. Assigning students a short reading list of articles during a clerkship is a helpful way to augment clinical education. Reading and discussing articles with their preceptors helps students learn about conditions or treatments they have not yet seen. Furthermore, it helps students, regardless of their chosen specialty, learn the skills to appraise clinical research and apply it to practice. To satisfy multiple educational goals, we have chosen a variety of article types. Landmark studies help students understand the clinical discovery process and the evidence base behind standard clinical practices. Review articles summarize a vast body of evidence for conditions and treatments that students may not often see. Finally, supplemental readings elicit thought and discussion about challenging psychiatric research and practice topics.

Landmark Articles

Lithium Salts in the Treatment of Psychotic Excitement

John Cade published a groundbreaking study describing the significant improvement of severe mania in chronic and recurrent cases with lithium salts. In the paper, Cade (1949) first reviewed the history of lithium use in medicine and the adverse effects that later limited its use. He detailed his experiments with guinea pigs that led him to choose lithium salts in the treatment of mania. Cade also described 10 male patients suffering from chronic or recurrent mania treated with lithium. Their manic states responded very well to the drug, effectively treating all but one case. A few patients were functioning well enough to return to work soon after initiating treatment. In one case, although lithium cured the man's mania, the side effects were intolerable. Treatment was discontinued, and the patient reverted to his previous manic state. Common adverse effects of lithium include gastrointestinal symptoms, such as nausea and abdominal pain, as well as neurological issues that can present as toxicity and even be fatal if medication is not withheld.

This article represents the first time a specific medication was shown to have a therapeutic effect on bipolar disorder. It has had a lasting impact on psychiatry and was essential to establishing lithium as a standard treatment for bipolar patients. Although much more has been learned about lithium and its benefits, risks, and dosing, Cade (1949) still provides an accurate overview of its efficacy and side effects while being quite interesting from a historical perspective.

Taking Care of the Hateful Patient

All physicians will encounter patients they experience as "difficult." A physician's adverse reactions to these patients can lead to unwanted health care outcomes and increase physician burnout. Groves (1978) reviewed countertransference toward four stereotypical complex patients. The article provides an opportunity for the educator to explore countertransference as a relevant concept for all physicians. It also helps students develop compassion for some challenging patients they may encounter and think about techniques to better treat different types of complex patients while avoiding burnout. Although the article offers little empirical evidence for its assertions, it encourages readers to examine their feelings—even ones that a physician may shudder to admit to—and channel those feelings in a fashion that can create a more productive physician–patient relationship.

Effectiveness of Antipsychotic Drugs in Patients With Chronic Schizophrenia

The CATIE (Clinical Antipsychotic Trials of Intervention Effectiveness) trial was an extensive study of more than 1,400 patients comparing the effectiveness, safety, and tolerability of antipsychotic drugs in the treatment of schizophrenia (Lieberman et al. 2005). Drugs studied over the 18 months included atypical antipsychotics, olanzapine, quetiapine, and risperidone, as well as a typical antipsychotic, perphenazine. All antipsychotics had high rates of discontinuation (64%–82%), primarily owing to side effects and lack of efficacy. Efficacy did not vary across treatment arms, with atypical antipsychotics having no better remission of symptoms than the typical antipsychotic studied. The results of CATIE highlighted the challenge of maintaining adherence to treatment in schizophrenia. It influenced clinical practice by stressing the importance of balancing treatment with side effects and encouraged an individualized approach to treatment in schizophrenia. It was a landmark study in the treatment of schizophrenia with which any psychiatry trainee should be familiar.

Evaluation of Outcomes With Citalopram for Depression Using Measurement-Based Care in STAR*D: Implications for Clinical Practice

Similar to CATIE, but for depression, the STAR*D (Sequenced Treatment Alternatives to Relieve Depression) trial was a large multilevel study by the National Institute of Mental Health that included more than 4,000 patients (Trivedi et al. 2006). Its objective was to compare the effectiveness of different treatments for major depressive disorder and provide a guide for the next step of treatment in patients with major depression, who did not fully respond to initial antidepressant therapy. The methods were designed to mimic real-world conditions, with minimal exclusion criteria (it included patients with comorbidities and treatment resistance), and allow for patient preference in an open-label design. If a patient's symptoms did not achieve remission after 12 weeks of the first treatment, they could move on to the next treatment arm, switch treatment entirely, or add an adjunctive treatment. Similarly, if symptoms did not remit after the second treatment, a third treatment arm had options to switch or add on treatment, followed by a fourth treatment arm for any subjects who continued to have significant depressive symptoms.

STAR*D was a landmark study in psychiatry. It demonstrated that response and remission rates are limited in the treatment of depression with medications, even with the addition of cognitive therapy. Only 67% of subjects who completed the study achieved remission, and there were diminishing returns with each subsequent trial of treatment. This study also showed that treatment for depression takes significant time. Additionally, there were no significant differences in efficacy between any of the treatment arms; however, with the choice given to patients and the high dropout rate, there was limited power to assess this well. Despite its limitations, STAR*D is still one of the most important studies in psychiatric pharmacology and a must-read for students.

Review Articles

The Placebo Effect in Psychiatric Practice

The placebo effect refers to improvements in a patient's condition due to positive beliefs and associations with the treatment rather than the treatment itself. The word *placebo* has long held negative connotations and associations with fake and unhelpful therapies. In recent years, however, much research across a variety of diseases has shown that placebo pills make changes to the body similar to those of their active pharmacologic counterparts. Because placebo treatment has its most significant impact on the subjective experience of an illness, such as pain and distress, it has a powerful effect on psychiatric illness. In many illnesses of depression and anxiety, patients improve almost as much with a placebo as they do with standard treatment. It is less effective for schizophrenia, major neurocognitive disorder, and obsessive-compulsive disorder.

Bernstein and Brown (2017) argued that understanding the placebo effect can enhance clinical practice by recognizing the power of patient expectations and integrating this awareness into treatment strategies. The power of a placebo is not just in taking a pill, but in the associated treatment situation. A psychiatrist's history-taking can provide reassurance, reduce distress, and instill hope. Not surprisingly, several studies show that a strong patient–doctor relationship is associated with improved outcomes. Patient expectations are another significant contributing factor. How a physician manages a patient's expectations in preparation for treatment undoubtedly affects how the patient responds. The authors also describe the potential for using placebo openly to get a conditioned response that may be very helpful in certain psychiatric illnesses, particularly substance use disorders, to treat successfully while using less medication.

We recommend this article, which explains the benefit of the placebo effect and encourages its use as a tool available to physicians. It is important that medical students, no matter what field they choose, understand that there are many different facets of treatments, besides the pill or procedure prescribed, that can contribute to the patient's healing.

How Important Are the Common Factors in Psychotherapy? An Update

Positive outcomes are seen in every popular psychotherapy modality. This result has led psychiatrists to wonder if there is something else, other than the particular treatment protocol involved, contributing to the patient's improvement. This has sparked a discussion of *common factors*, or the elements shared across different psychotherapeutic approaches, contributing to positive treatment effects. Wampold (2015) reviewed known common factors, described evidence for their impact, and placed them within the contextual model to show how these factors can lead to positive change.

The author reviewed meta-analyses to determine the effect sizes of common factors and specific factors in psychotherapy: goal consensus between therapist and patient, empathy expressed, treatment alliance, positive regard, individual therapist, congruence, cultural adaptation, and expectations, among others. Goal consensus and empathy have the most substantial effect sizes; alliance, positive regard, and individual therapist have moderate effects. Each of these individually have more significant effect sizes than the noncommon (or specific) therapy factors, which have modest effects on outcome. The authors explained each factor and the evidence behind its benefits.

There is a tendency to focus on how one psychotherapeutic approach is better than another, but evidence shows that we can attribute most of the benefit of any approach to the qualities of the therapist and elements common to all psychotherapies. It is important to understand this when learning about psychotherapy. Additionally, medical students benefit from appreciating the importance of their patient interactions and the potential difference they can make. The empathy they show, the trust they build, and the goals and expectations they set can make positive changes in their patients.

Electroconvulsive Therapy for Depression

Electroconvulsive therapy (ECT) remains one of psychiatry's most potent and controversial tools. Unfortunately, many students do not observe ECT, and without a proper understanding of the facts, misconceptions about ECT can persist. In this paper, Lisanby (2007) presented a patient with psychotic depression, a typical case encountered in the inpatient psychiatric setting. She succinctly described the procedure, which is particularly helpful for students who may not be able to see many ECT cases. The author also discussed the impact of depression and the remission rates of conventional treatments, which highlight the need for alternative therapeutic modalities, such as ECT. The pathophysiology of depression was reviewed, as well as some of the procedure's mechanisms of action, which are helpful educational points for a student in clinical training. The paper also discussed the evidence for ECT and some areas where questions remain. The side effects of ECT are described, with a particular focus on cognitive side effects, one of the largest areas of concern for patients and clinicians. Education regarding electroconvulsive therapy remains important so that physicians can recommend this potentially lifesaving treatment.

Neurobiological Advances From the Brain Disease Model of Addiction

Addictions have a significant impact on health and will be encountered by nearly all physicians in their professional lives, and often in their personal lives. Volkow et al. (2016) explained how drug addictions change the neurobiology of a person. Understanding the neurobiology of addiction can help a physician understand the struggles of a patient with addiction and decrease stigma. The article highlighted the neurobiology behind many of the behaviors medical students will observe when treating a patient with addiction. It describes the neurobiology behind the reward system, the so-called anti-reward system, and brain dysregulations that can lead to impulsive choices. The article also explains why certain people, places, things, or situations can trigger cravings, even in those who have long been sober. Many students wonder why patients do not seem to want to stop using substances or repeatedly relapse, despite adverse consequences. The article briefly touches on why some people tend to develop addictions and explains how knowledge of these neurobiological changes guides treatment, although it does not discuss treatment strategies in depth. It also eloquently shows how understanding the neurobiology of addiction can influence public health policy. By understanding the neurobiological changes that addiction brings, the reader can develop increased compassion for a person who has a drug addiction and is having difficulties achieving and maintaining sobriety.

Thought-Provoking Articles

Suicide From the Golden Gate Bridge

Since its construction in 1937, the Golden Gate Bridge in San Francisco Bay has been one of the most popular locations in the world for suicide. Blaustein and Fleming (2009) presented three clinical vignettes of individuals who died by suicide by jumping from the Golden Gate Bridge. In doing so, the authors emphasized the problem of suicide and the diversity of those who die by suicide. The paper also identified suicide as an often-impulsive act and argues that removing easy access to something strongly associated with suicide does more than displace the behavior—it can reduce its overall occurrence. The authors advocated for the construction of a barrier at the Golden Gate Bridge to reduce suicide in the Bay Area.

This article calls attention to the importance of suicide as a public health issue and the need for preventive measures. It also cites many examples in the literature to refute a common but mistaken belief that those who die by suicide are determined and that simple obstacles cannot save them. In fact, removing easy access to lethal means is very effective in reducing suicide risk. This fact is important for physicians, especially psychiatrists or psychiatric trainees, to understand. On January 1, 2024, thanks in part to this paper, a suicide barrier was installed on both sides of the Golden Gate Bridge. Since then, "early evidence indicates the installation of safety nets on the Golden Gate Bridge is associated with an immediate and substantial reduction in suicides at the site" (Shin et al. 2025).

No Health Without Mental Health

Most students will not elect for a career in psychiatry. However, all students will see patients with psychiatric illnesses and those illnesses affect the patient's general medical health. Many physicians may not be aware that mental disorders are among the most significant contributors to global disease burden, morbidity, and mortality. Prince et al. (2007) reviewed the ways in which mental disorders affect medical conditions such as cardiovascular disease, diabetes, and communicable diseases. In addition, the authors described how maternal mental health can impact a child's well-being, offering educators an opportunity to discuss the impact of upbringing in shaping health. They also emphasized the influence of broader societal issues, including gender disparities, poverty, and violence, on health. Finally, the authors discussed how changes in public health policy can improve health outcomes. This paper highlights the importance of mental health literacy for all physicians and illustrates how clinicians can advocate for societal and public health changes to improve overall health.

Identifying Articles That Are Likely to Have a High Impact

The total number of articles continues to increase every day. One bibliographical analysis found that more than 80,000 psychiatric articles were published between 2011 and 2015, with the rate of new articles increasing during those years (Zhang et al. 2017). Given the rate of publication, keeping up with the literature can be an overwhelming prospect. For the medical teacher, it takes great skill to choose articles that will have lasting value. The articles suggested here represent a starting point, but the field is changing rapidly and many articles on the list with time will become obsolete.

Most teachers start with a database (e.g., PubMed, PsycINFO, or Scopus). In each case, they should familiarize themselves with filters, such as "review article," "systematic review," or "meta-analysis," to locate high-impact papers that synthesize existing research. Most will prioritize articles published in well-regarded journals—such as *The American Journal of Psychiatry*, *JAMA Psychiatry*, and *The British Journal of Psychiatry*—as these tend to publish rigorous and influential work. An article's citation count can also signal its impact, although newer, yet groundbreaking, studies may not have many citations yet.

Beyond database metrics, one should consider the author's institutional affiliation and history of contributions to the field. It helps to pay attention to articles widely discussed at conferences, in professional newsletters, or on social media platforms, which increasingly spotlight emerging work. Reading editorials, commentaries, or journal highlights can also help in recognizing key developments.

Secondary sources may also help identify important articles. Many societies and organizations publish lists of the most important articles of the year in their fields. For example, the Academy of Consultation-Liaison Psychiatry uses a structured method that considers the importance of the article's subject, conclusions, and the quality of the methodology, to identify the top consultation-liaison articles in a given year (Simpson et al. 2021).

Conclusions

Students have access to countless articles and books to complement their clinical education, but it can be overwhelming to sort through these on their own and self-assign appropriate materials. Providing a short reading list during the psychiatry clerkship is a fairly easy and helpful way for a facilitator to supplement discussion and learning on the rotation. The list can be adjusted based on the educator's preferences and specific points they would like to prioritize during the rotation. Additional papers can also be offered case-by-case, according to the student's specific interests.

Key Points

- Assigning students a predetermined short list of articles is a helpful way to augment clinical education during a clerkship.
- Additional papers can be offered case-by-case, according to the students' specific interests.

References

Bernstein MH, Brown WA: The placebo effect in psychiatric practice. Curr Psychiatr 16(11):29–34, 2017 29910696

Blaustein M, Fleming A: Suicide from the Golden Gate Bridge. Am J Psychiatry 166(10):1111–1116, 2009 19797444

Cade JFJ: Lithium salts in the treatment of psychotic excitement. Med J Aust 2(10):349–352, 1949 18142718

Groves JE: Taking care of the hateful patient. N Engl J Med 298(16):883–887, 1978 634331

Lieberman JA, Stroup TS, McEvoy JP, et al; Clinical Antipsychotic Trials of Intervention Effectiveness (CATIE) Investigators: Effectiveness of antipsychotic drugs in patients with chronic schizophrenia. N Engl J Med 353(12):1209–1223, 2005 16172203

Lisanby SH: Electroconvulsive therapy for depression. N Engl J Med 357(19):1939–1945, 2007 17989386

Prince M, Patel V, Saxena S, et al: No health without mental health. Lancet 370(9590):859–877, 2007 17804063

Shin S, Pirkis J, Clapperton A, Spittal M: Change in suicides during and after the installation of barriers at the Golden Gate Bridge. Inj Prev ip-2024-045604, 2025 40101955

Simpson SA, Bienvenu OJ, Andrews SR, et al: Identifying the most important consultation-liaison psychiatry publications in 2020 using a novel literature assessment instrument. J Acad Consult Liaison Psychiatry 62(5):493–500, 2021 34048960

Trivedi MH, Rush AJ, Wisniewski SR, et al; STAR*D Study Team: Evaluation of outcomes with citalopram for depression using measurement-based care in STAR*D: implications for clinical practice. Am J Psychiatry 163(1):28–40, 2006 16390886

Volkow ND, Koob GF, McLellan AT: Neurobiologic advances from the brain disease model of addiction. N Engl J Med 374(4):363–371, 2016 26816013

Wampold BE: How important are the common factors in psychotherapy? An update. World Psychiatry 14(3):270–277, 2015 26407772

Zhang J, Chen X, Gao X, et al: Worldwide research productivity in the field of psychiatry. Int J Ment Health Syst 11:20, 2017 28289438

14

The Art of a Good Presentation in Psychiatry: Teaching Techniques and Slide Preparation

Carlyle H. Chan, M.D.

Although the current emphasis in education is on active learning techniques (flipped classroom, case-based learning, etc.) (French et al. 2020; Padmanabha et al. 2023), the traditional passive mode of lecturing remains a dominant vehicle for disseminating information, particularly to a large audience. Certain strategies can prove useful when preparing a lecture. These can be divided into three categories: reflection, augmentation, and delivery.

Reflection

During the process of reflection, one needs to consider what to cover, who the audience is, and, perhaps most importantly, what the audience should learn. To communicate the take-home points, think about how to convey the information—and whether a lecture is even necessary.

It is important to ask how best to facilitate learning. Another consideration is how your audience might learn in relation to what you are trying to teach. According to the 1885 Ebbinghaus forgetting curve (since replicated) (Murre and Dros 2015), learners will not retain much of what they learned after several days. Therefore, a data dump may be an efficient way for a speaker to convey information, but it is an ineffective vehicle for retention and learning. For example, when I was asked to deliver a lecture on resident mental health and mental health services to residents in each of the institution's residency programs, I quickly found a disinterested audience. When I changed the format to a Jeopardy!-style game, residents became competitively involved, with one resident spontaneously approaching me afterward to say, "I remember the phone number for resident mental health."

Several studies have suggested ways to improve the retention of lecture material, including short-duration didactic lectures, audience response devices (Cain 2008), use of videos, and open discussions (Pasquale and Pugnaire 2002; Soriano et al. 2010). Medical schools have found that frequent quizzes enhance student learning (Cook and Babon 2017; Dengri et al. 2021). A prelecture quiz can introduce the subject matter and prime the audience to listen more intently for answers. A postlecture quiz reinforces retention by applying the content just provided. Even answering incorrectly can be beneficial (we tend to recall wrong answers longer than right ones). All of these are attempts to incorporate more active learning experiences into a lecture rather than the usual passive transfer of knowledge.

It is also important to recognize the background of the intended audience. A lecture to the public could be quite different than one addressed to colleagues—professional terminology would need to be clarified, for instance.

Just as film directors use a storyboard to plan movie scenes, planning the direction and sequence of your presentation can help you visualize, guide, and arrange the flow of your material (Peck 2023). Analog methods (3-by-5-inch index cards) or a digital draft in PowerPoint can assist in accomplishing this task. In PowerPoint, the "slide sorter" view helps when moving slides around. Taking time to plan how to make a lecture more compelling and engaging will aid the audience in retaining more of the information you provide.

Augmentation

The second strategic category is augmentation. When constructing slides, consider whether the slides will augment (or supplement) your speaking points or whether the slides will distract and detract from your presentation. The Internet is replete with examples of how slides can take away from the speaker's message and bore the audience—a common expression these days is "death by PowerPoint."

The most common mistake is placing too much information on a single slide. A slide that is word-heavy, contains too many bullet points, or features graphs or tables that are too small or overly complicated impedes audience understanding. During the official examination of the 2003 Columbia Shuttle Craft disaster by NASA's Accident Investigation Board, such an error was found to have led to an unfortunate literal example of death by PowerPoint (Figure 14.1). When the underbody of the craft was struck on takeoff by a piece of foam insulation, engineers hurriedly studied and prepared a safety report to determine whether the spacecraft was safe to return to Earth at the mission's end. They delivered the report through PowerPoint presentations. It turned out that important information was buried under subheadings and levels of information on a slide; the result was the disastrous disintegration of the shuttle upon reentry. The board concluded that reports should be submitted via Microsoft Word, not PowerPoint (Columbia Accident Investigation Board 2003).

Edward Tufte, Yale Professor Emeritus, was a member of that investigation board. A paper on his website, "PowerPoint Does Rocket Science" (Tufte 2005), displays one of the NASA PowerPoint slides and describes in detail how the meaning of the slide got buried.

All too often, we hear a speaker say, "I know you can't read this, but…". To improve readability and declutter a slide, one method is the *1-7-7 rule* (Reynolds 2011). Each slide should have only one point. There should be a maximum of seven lines, with a maximum of seven words per line. Other combinations of points, lines, and words are easily found on the internet (e.g., 1-8-8, 1-6-6, and 1-5-5). Even following these guidelines, though, can result in a word-heavy slide.

To simplify content, there are also schools of even more conservative (or perhaps more radical) perspectives. These include the Kawasaki, Takahashi, and Lessig methods. The common feature in all three styles is the need to simplify your slides and presentations and to use more visual images in conveying your message. The Kawasaki method proposes a limit of 10 slides, 20-minute duration, and 30-point type (Kawasaki 2005). The Takahashi method advocates using only one word or idea per slide (as Thoreau said, "Simplify, simplify") in the largest font possible (Presentation Zen 2005). The Lessig method borrows from Takahashi in using few words on a slide but makes generous use of photos, graphics,

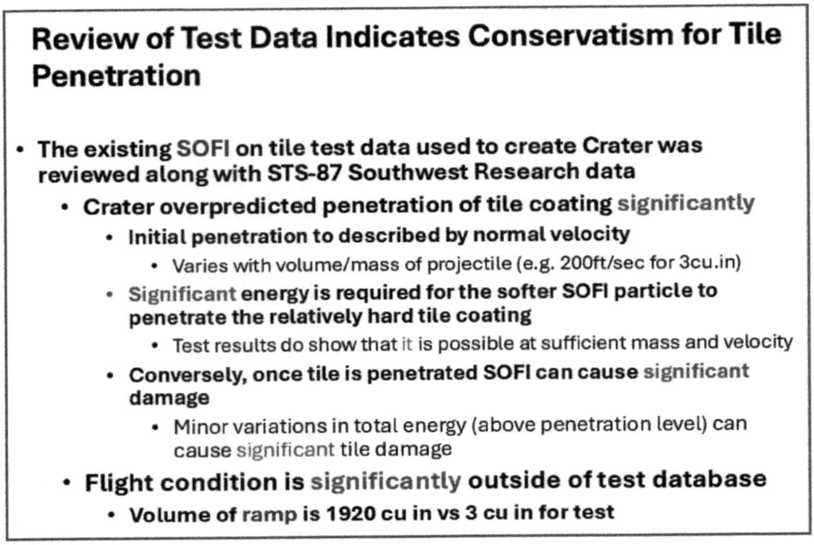

Figure 14.1 Example of standard PowerPoint format.

Source. Columbia Accident Investigation Board 2003; public domain.

Performance data about the space shuttle in a PowerPoint slide, showing how the default style can make it difficult to recognize critical data. Tufte (2005) pointed out that, among other problems, the slide contained an inaccurate summary statement, used six different levels of bullets, and relegated the most important point (that existing data were not relevant to a craft of Columbia's size) to the lowest-hierarchy and smallest bullet point. (Some black text on the slide is gray to highlight possible sources of problems.)

and video clips, which are shown rapidly. One such presentation was conducted 15 minutes while displaying hundreds of slides (Dlugan 2007).

If you display all the bullet points simultaneously, the audience generally reads faster than you can speak, which can diminish the audience's capacity to focus on what you have just said. To avoid this, decrease the material on each slide, using multiple slides with one (bullet) point on each slide. Alternatively, use the animation function, which allows you to stage your bullet points (if you are still using them). Each point will appear as you progress through the slide, keeping your audience's attention on the point you're speaking to. (A word of caution: PowerPoint has multiple ways of animating a bullet point—swirling, twisting, splitting, spinning, growing, shrinking—all of which can be distracting. It is best to stick with the "appear" option.) To keep focus

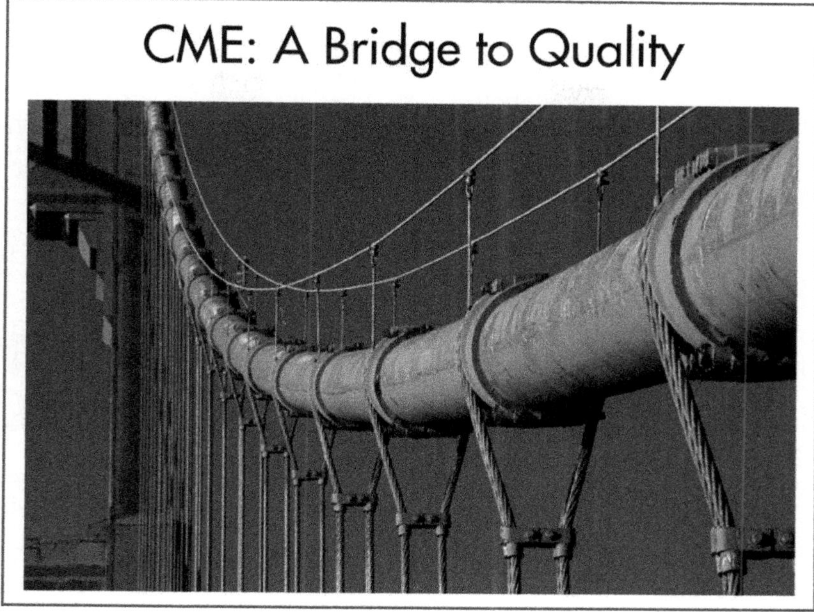

Figure 14.2 PowerPoint generally defaults to a smaller rectangle within the slide...

on the current talking point, you can also fade a bullet point once you have completed it.

It has been said that a picture is worth a thousand words. Introducing photographs or other images (including video) into a presentation can break up the monotony of printed words and add visuals to reinforce your topic. PowerPoint's insert feature for photos and videos places them in a box in the middle of the slide, allowing you to write a caption or title above or below the image (Figure 14.2). Blank space surrounding the image is wasted space that conveys no information, so after inserting a photo or video, you may enlarge it by clicking on the corner of the image and pulling it diagonally to fill the entire slide. Then, you may overlap a text box onto the image in a contrasting color (Figure 14.3).

Of course, do be sure your image is of sufficient resolution to remain sharp when expanded. (You will know it is not if the photo becomes pixelated.)

When using photos or graphs that are not yours, pay attention to copyright. "Fair use" might apply if you're addressing a small group

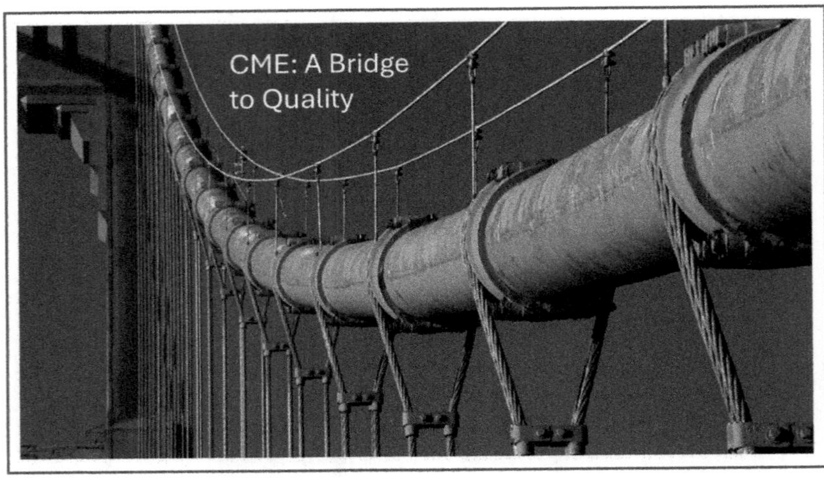

Figure 14.3 ... but it is easy to increase the image size, increasing the dramatic effect.

or class, but when giving lectures to larger audiences or posting slides online, you must respect permission and copyright terms. To avoid copyright violations, use original photographs or images, purchase stock photos, or use photos in the public domain. Alternatively, use items shared on Creative Commons (search.creativecommons.org or commons.wikimedia.org), which you may use with proper attribution (Creative Commons 2019). Figure 14.4 shows the kind of photographs available to illustrate the concepts you're discussing.

Another choice you will make for your slides is the font to use. Three decisions are involved when considering fonts: type, color, and size. Data suggest that sans serif fonts are more accessible for audiences to read (Schultz 2009). Second, when preparing a presentation on a computer, remember that the screen is backlit; thus, colors are much more vivid and saturated than when projected onto a screen by an LCD projector. Hence, some color combinations can appear washed out. Choose colors that provide sufficient contrast, and don't be afraid to just use black and white. Third, font size does matter. The typical default size is 32 points, but even this can be difficult to view from a distance (Figure 14.5).

Displaying a graph or chart like those used in a textbook presents some additional challenges. Figures in a textbook are usually accompanied by a detailed explanation, allowing the reader to move back

Dreyfus Model:
Developmental stages of learning

- Novice
- Advanced beginner
- Competent
- Proficient
- Expert

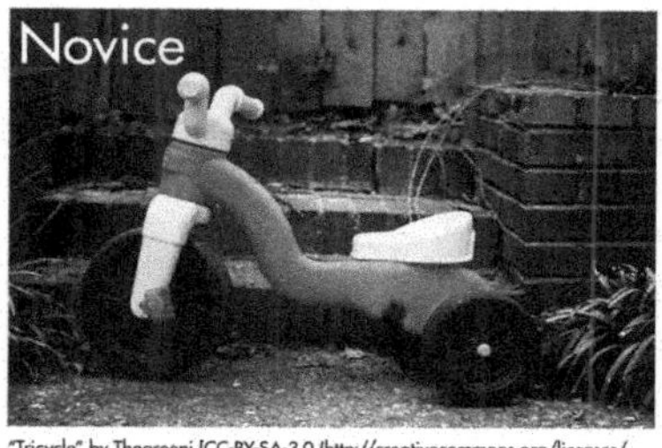

"Tricycle" by Thegreenj [CC-BY-SA-3.0 (http://creativecommons.org/licenses/by-sa/3.0)], via Wikimedia Commons. Available at: https://upload.wikimedia.org/wikipedia/commons/1/11/SelectivelyeditedTricycle.jpg

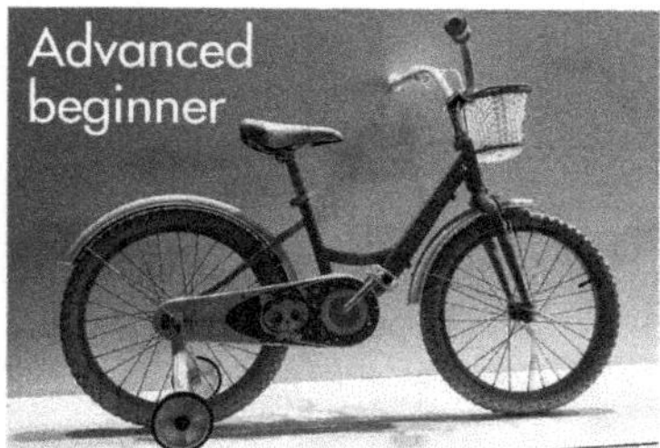

"Suncross Sweetie, Eurobike 2024, Frankfurt am Main" by Matti Blume [CC-BY-SA-3.0], via Wikimedia Commons. Available at: https://commons.wikimedia.org/wiki/File:Suncross_Sweetie,_Eurobike_2024,_Frankfurt_am_Main_(EB245525).jpg

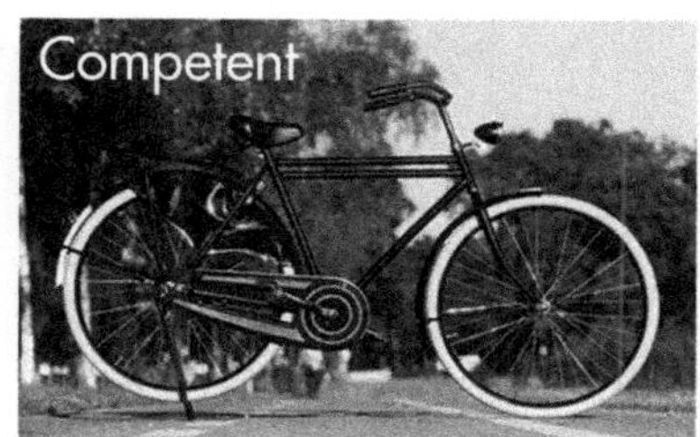

"Dutch bicycle" by Petar Milošević [CC-BY-SA-3.0 (http://creativecommons.org/licenses/by-sa/3.0)], via Wikimedia Commons. Available at: https://upload.wikimedia.org/wikipedia/commons/b/bc/Dutch_bicycle.jpg

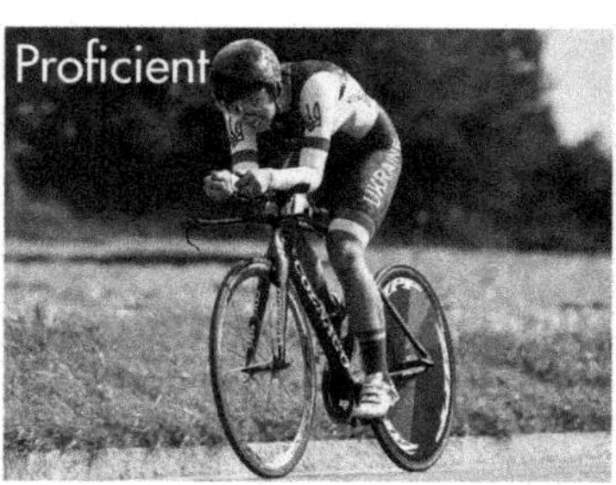

"2018 UCI Road World Championships Innsbruck Women Juniors ITT Tetyana Yaschenko (UKR)" by Granada [CC-BY-SA-3.0], via Wikimedia Commons. Available at: https://upload.wikimedia.org/wikipedia/commons/9/96/20180924_UCI_Road_World_Championships_Innsbruck_Women_Juniors_ITT_Tetyana_Yaschenko_%28UKR%29_DSC_7564.jpg

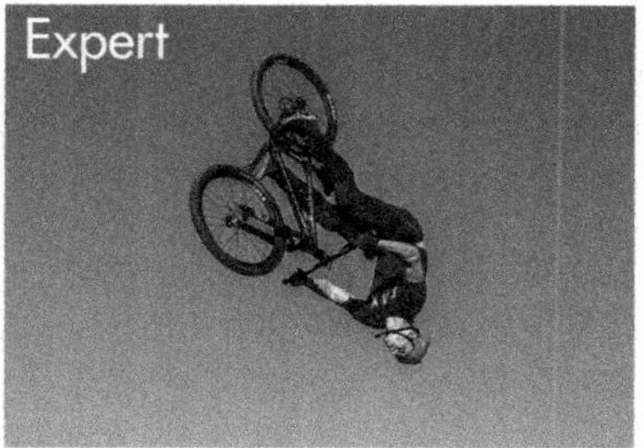

"Dirt Jump" by Fischer.H [CC-BY-SA-3.0], via Wikimedia Commons. Available at: https://upload.wikimedia.org/wikipedia/commons/c/cc/Dirt_Bike_IMG_4202.jpg

Figure 14.4 **An example series of slides demonstrating the Dreyfus skill model: the first slide uses text to simply list the stages, whereas the subsequent slides graphically demonstrate metaphors for each step.**

Source. Printed in figure.

and forth from the figure to the text to better understand the significance. Audiences don't have that option when viewing a presenter's slide. Presenting a complicated graph or table requires time to orient

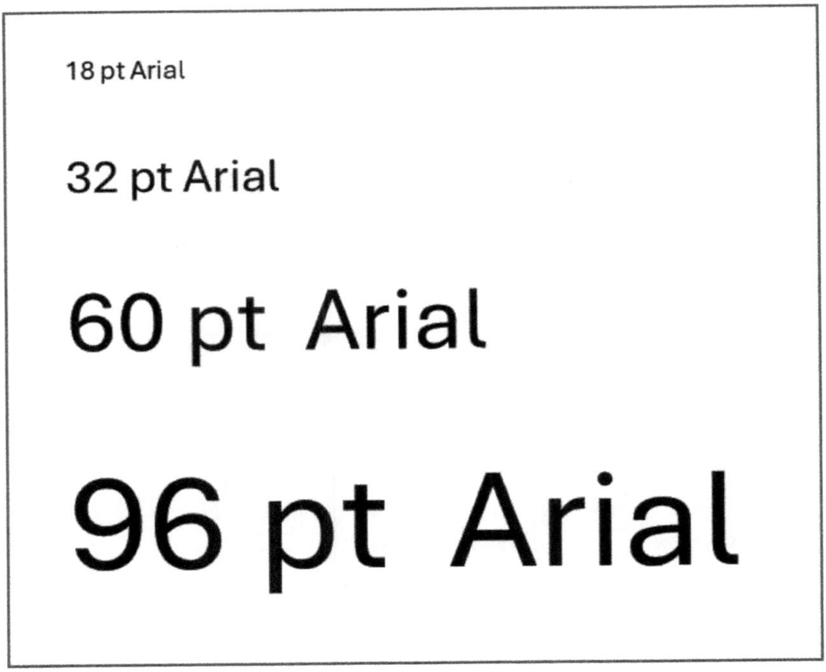

18 pt Arial

32 pt Arial

60 pt Arial

96 pt Arial

Figure 14.5 Readability of different font sizes.

and explain. Also, if the graph or chart is complex, it may be difficult to view from the back of the room. In some cases, such a slide might require the bulk of a presentation to review. Enlargement of specific regions of the graph or chart might also be helpful in elucidating the intricacies of a complex graph or chart.

Delivery

Viewing a lecture as a performance can bring on performance anxiety, but it is necessary to decide how best to deliver the talk. The first rule of thumb: do not write your talk on slides and then read them aloud.

Years ago, educational researchers articulated what has come to be called the Dr. Fox Effect. An actor, introduced as Dr. Fox, gave a prepared speech to a medical audience. It was presented in a light, engaging, and humorous manner. The talk was met with positive reviews.

Crucially, the presentation contained absolutely no factual material (experimenter63 2011; Naftulin et al. 1973).

Rather than concluding that style was everything, researchers conducted a second experiment (Ware and Williams 1975). They prepared six talks on the "Biochemistry of Learning." Two of the presentations contained 26 facts each, two had 14 facts, and two had only 4 facts. One set of three talks (with 26, 14, and 4 facts) was presented in what they called a "low seduction" style of delivery—a dull monotone. A second set of the three talks was delivered in a "high seduction" manner—with enthusiasm, engagement, and humor. A quiz based on all 26 facts was administered at the end of each presentation.

As expected, audience members in both groups (low and high seduction) who heard more facts generally did better on the quiz than listeners who heard fewer facts. What was surprising was that members of the high-seduction, low-facts subgroup generally did about as well on the quiz as members of the low-seduction, high-facts subgroup. This experiment gave credence to the perspective that delivery style can influence the retention of spoken words. Having some passion for your subject material is essential and that interest and enthusiasm can elevate your presentation beyond a monotone. Evidence also shows that the human brain is more receptive to remembering a story than a list. Narrating a story or finding ways to weave in anecdotes can assist an audience in retaining your talking points (Easton 2016).

Another aspect of viewing lectures as a performance is stage presence. It may be useful to move away from the podium and walk among your listeners, particularly with smaller audiences. Doing so eliminates a physical barrier (the podium) to better engage the audience (Scientifica n.d.). Making eye contact is helpful. Focus on one individual in the audience to deliver one point before moving on to the next person and the next point to be made (Inc. 2014).

Broadcast journalists take courses on speaking before a camera. They learn to modulate their voices so as not to speak in a monotone (Toastmasters International 2011). They pay attention to vocalized pauses, remembering not to insert "er" or "uh" while thinking of what to say next (Cohen 2012; Inc. 2014). News announcers also remember to slow their speech rate to a conversational speed.

Verbalized transitions can be useful in a presentation. A journal article contains printed transitions (introduction, methods, results, discussion), but such markers can be missing in a talk. The common adage, "Tell them what you're going tell them. Tell them. Then tell them what you told them," remains useful. Once you say "in summary" or "in conclusion," don't drone on and on. Be aware and respectful of time limits. In addition, students typically respond attentively to hearing, "This next point will be on the exam."

Avoid slide text dissociation (not having a slide for the point you are addressing). Should this circumstance arise, in PowerPoint, you can press the B key on the keyboard to turn the screen black; pressing it again will return you to your previous slide. Similarly, pressing the W key will toggle the screen to white and back again.

Another common adage, "How do you get to Carnegie Hall? Practice, practice, practice" applies to presenting. It is important to rehearse your talk to familiarize yourself with the material and the timing. In the event of a technical meltdown, you should be ready to carry on despite the lack of slides.

Tips for Success

Some final takeaways:

- If delivering a talk in person, arrive early. There may not be a parking space nearby.
- Check out the venue where you will be speaking and inspect the room size and whether you will need amplification; if so, perform a microphone sound check. If there is no microphone, ensure you can project your voice to the back of the room.
- If presenting virtually, it is wise to connect early to have time to test both sound and share-screen capability in advance.
- Regarding handouts: It has become customary for organizers to request a copy of your slide deck to load on their projecting computer or print out for attendees. If using photographs or videos, you may find that the file size is too large to attach to an email. A cloud storage transfer service such as Dropbox or OneDrive may be necessary to transmit your slides.
- Typically, only a small percentage of attendees actually review handouts provided at a conference. In keeping with the suggestion of keeping text minimal, consider omitting the slide handouts. A written version of the talk or a related paper might be a more useful handout.
- A resource for role models in presentation skills are TED talks (https://www.ted.com/). These are short, informative, highly rehearsed, and polished presentations that engage an audience's attention.

- Another speaker resource is Garr Reynold's *Presentation Zen,* which expands on techniques for simplifying slide construction (Reynolds 2011).

Conclusions

Reflection, augmentation, and delivery are three strategies that can assist in producing a professionally appearing presentation that will both capture your audience's attention and assist them in retaining the information you provide.

Key Points

- Despite the current emphasis on active learning techniques in medical education, the traditional passive mode of lecturing remains a dominant vehicle for disseminating information, particularly to a large audience.
- Certain strategies can prove useful when preparing and delivering a lecture, aiming at making a presentation more engaging and facilitating learning.

References

Cain J, Robinson E: A primer on audience response systems: current applications and future considerations. Am J Pharm Educ 52940:77, 2008

Cohen SD: Tips on Public Speaking: Eliminating the Dreaded "Um." Harvard Extension School, 2012. Available at: https://extension.harvard.edu/blog/tips-on-public-speaking-eliminating-the-dreaded-um/. Accessed October 14, 2024.

Columbia Accident Investigation Board. The CAIB Report—Volume I. Columbia Accident Investigation Board, August 2003. Available at: https://govinfo.library.unt.edu/caib/news/report/pdf/vol1/full/caib_report_volume1.pdf. Accessed June 16, 2025.

Cook BR, Babon A: Active learning through online quizzes: better learning and less (busy) work. J Geogr High Educ 41:24–38, 2017

Creative Commons. About CC Licenses. Creative Commons, 2019. Available at: https://creativecommons.org/share-your-work/cclicenses/. Accessed October 14, 2024.

Dengri C, Gill A, Chopra J, et al: A review of the quiz, as a new dimension in medical education. Cureus 13(10):e18854, 2021 34804707

Dlugan A: Critique: Lessig Method Presentation Style (Dick Hardt, Identity 2.0, OSCON 2005). Six Minutes, 2007. Available at: https://sixminutes.dlugan.com/tag/lessig-method/. Accessed October 14, 2024.

Easton G: How medical teachers use narratives in lectures: a qualitative study. BMC Med Educ 16:3, 2016 26742778

experimenter63. The Dr Fox Lecture. experimenter63, June 13, 2011. Available at: https://www.youtube.com/watch?v=RcxW6nrWwtc. Accessed October 14, 2024.

French H, Arias-Shah A, Gisondo C, Gray MM: Perspectives: the flipped classroom in graduate medical education. Neoreviews 21(3):e150–e156, 2020 32123119

Inc. 10 Reasons Eye Contact Is Everything in Public Speaking. Inc., 2014. Available at: https://www.inc.com/sims-wyeth/10-reasons-why-eye-contact-can-change-peoples-perception-of-you.html. Accessed October 14, 2024.

Kawasaki G: The 10/20/30 Rule of PowerPoint. Guy Kawasaki, December 30, 2005. Available at: https://guykawasaki.com/the_102030_rule/. Accessed October 14, 2024.

Murre JMJ, Dros J: Replication and analysis of Ebbinghaus' forgetting curve. PLoS One 10(7):e0120644, 2015 26148023

Naftulin DH, Ware JE Jr, Donnelly FA: The Doctor Fox Lecture: a paradigm of educational seduction. J Med Educ 48(7):630–635, 1973 4708420

Padmanabha TS, Shilpashree YD, Ajay N, et al: Is there a case for case-based learning in pharmacology? Cureus 15(6):e39835, 2023 37397677

Pasquale SJ, Pugnaire MP: Preparing medical students to teach. Acad Med 77(11):1175–1176, 2002 12431958

Peck D: How to Create a Storyboard for e-Learning (Instructional Design), May 2023. Available at: https://www.devlinpeck.com/content/create-storyboard-for-elearning. Accessed July 14, 2025.

Presentation Zen: Living large: "Takahashi Method" uses king-sized text as a visual. Presentation Zen, 2005. Available at: https://www.presentationzen.com/presentationzen/2005/09/living_large_ta.html. Accessed October 14, 2024.

Reynolds G: Presentation Zen: Simple Ideas on Presentation Design and Delivery. Indianapolis, New Riders, 2011

Schultz DM: Why you should use sans serif fonts for figures, posters, and slides. Eloquent Science, 2009. Available at: https://eloquentscience.com/2009/09/why-you-should-use-sans-serif-fonts-for-figures-posters-and-slides/. Accessed October 14, 2024.

Scientifica: 9 simple and effective public speaking tips for scientists. Scientifica, n.d. Available at: https://www.scientifica.uk.com/neurowire/9-simple-and-effective-public-speaking-tips-for-scientists. Accessed October 14, 2024.

Soriano RP, Blatt B, Coplit L, et al: Teaching medical students how to teach: a national survey of students-as-teachers programs in U.S. medical schools. Acad Med 85(11):1725–1731, 2010 20881824

Toastmasters International: Your Speaking Voice: Tips for Adding Strength and Authority to Your Voice. Toastmasters International, 2011. Available at: https://ccdn.toastmasters.org/medias/files/department-documents/education-documents/199-your-speaking-voice.pdf. Accessed October 14, 2024.

Tufte E: PowerPoint Does Rocket Science—and Better Techniques for Technical Reports. The Work of Edward Tufte and Graphics Press, 2005. Available at: https://www.edwardtufte.com/notebook/powerpoint-does-rocket-science-and-better-techniques-for-technical-reports/. Accessed October 14, 2024.

Ware JE Jr, Williams RG: The Dr. Fox effect: a study of lecturer effectiveness and ratings of instruction. J Med Educ 50(2):149–156, 1975 1120118

15

Beyond Lecturing

Flipped Classroom, Problem-Based Learning, and Other Active Learning Strategies to Teach Psychiatry

Sindhu A. Idicula, M.D.
Vivian Wang, M.D.
Laura Kenyon, M.D.

Lecture-based teaching, the traditional approach in undergraduate medical education, is fraught with significant limitations. Lectures encourage students to listen passively, limiting their ability to engage with or process the material. Their learning results from note-taking and memorization rather than applying and critically assessing material (King 1993).

The field of psychiatry evolves daily. Without building the skills to acquire knowledge quickly and appraise material critically, students are inadequately prepared for a clinical environment that rapidly shifts with the newest research. In addition, the practice of psychiatry is not simply a regurgitation of memorized material. It involves complex interpersonal skills, the ability to think through a nuanced differential diagnosis from information acquired in the clinical encounter, and effective work within the context of interdisciplinary teams to care for patients (Sandrone et al. 2020).

The field of education has shifted significantly over the past several decades, and pedagogical approaches that rely on active learning have been piloted and demonstrated to be successful in undergraduate medical education. These approaches, in contrast to lecture-based modalities, empower students to be active within their education, ask the questions relevant to solving real-world clinical problems, practice skills in finding answers to those questions within the evolving literature, and use each other as team members to help facilitate that process (Sandrone et al. 2020).

Overview of Strategies for Active Learning

Flipped Classroom

The flipped classroom (or backward classroom) is a model in which foundational concepts are provided to students before class so that class time is dedicated to building on fundamental concepts with higher-order learning (Persky and McLaughlin 2017).

The key elements to building a flipped classroom include

1. Preclass activity
2. In-class discussion and application
3. After-class activity

Preclass assignments present foundational material in preparation for an extension of learning in class. Materials may vary as to media, including textbook or literature reading, videos, narrated PowerPoints, web-based modules, or podcasts. When choosing materials for the preclass activity, care should be taken to ensure materials are available early, efficient in their content delivery, and at a developmentally appropriate level for the learners (Hurtubise et al. 2015).

Students engage in active application and problem-solving in class, reinforcing and extending the basic concepts learned before class.

Application exercises may take many forms, such as case vignettes, student or group presentations, think-pair-share, or role-playing. The instructor scaffolds the learners and helps them transition from basic concepts to more complex applications. They may point out links between preclass work and the in-class application, but must refrain from lecturing on the same material assigned preclass, which would eliminate the incentive for students to come prepared to class and may make students more passive in learning (Persky and McLaughlin 2017).

After class, the students engage in an after-class activity, reinforcing course objectives and integrating the material learned. After-class activities can include additional practice (as in class), slowly building complexity and mastery over time. Key factors in the after-class activity include timing (spacing to optimize knowledge retention) and diversity (increasing the transferability of the material to future coursework). After-class work also allows learners and teachers to assess mastery of the material.

Flipped classroom models have some significant advantages, such as promoting student engagement in the classroom. Students benefit from learning at their own pace in a self-directed model, allowing those who need it more time to process crucial concepts without being left behind in the classroom. Because most of the content is offloaded to preclass studying, class time can be dedicated to the complex and practical application of knowledge. This scaffolding principle is critical to the development of expertise and complex problem-solving. In addition, the flipped classroom fosters collaboration skills and self-awareness. Working with peers during the in-class activity provides the benefit of diverse perspectives and insights, and teachers have expanded opportunities to assess students' learning (Persky and McLaughlin 2017).

Some barriers to adopting a flipped classroom model include student and faculty time resources. The model requires considerable student preparatory time outside of class. The recommended ratio of time in-class and out-of-class (including prework and postwork) is 1:2, which may require attention to the academic workload for students. The success and efficacy of this model hinges on preparation, so that learners make the most of the in-class activity. Ways to foster learner accountability include embedding self-assessment or study guide questions in the preclass activity and setting clear expectations and objectives about preclass activities. Faculty time is also considerable in developing the initial curriculum and faculty development to effectively deliver a flipped classroom experience (Persky and McLaughlin 2017).

Case-Based Learning and Problem-Based Learning

Case-based learning (CBL) and problem-based learning (PBL) overlap in their strategies, but each methodology has distinctions that may make it suitable for various situations. Here we review each modality, then compare the two.

Case-Based Learning

CBL is a learner-centric approach in which students work in small groups (6–10 students) guided by a facilitator. They are presented with authentic clinical cases and work collaboratively to answer corresponding trigger questions designed to follow discrete learning objectives (McLean 2016; Thistlethwaite et al. 2012).

The CBL process involves the following:

1. Students review foundational knowledge before class.
2. Small groups are presented with cases for review.
3. Students collaboratively work through corresponding trigger questions.
4. Students return to large groups and discuss cases and trigger questions.
5. The facilitator guides discussion and teaching to ensure that students meet the learning objectives.

Ideal cases are based on real-world examples, use a storytelling style, and involve common scenarios that are widely applicable and aligned with the defined learning objectives. Using patient quotations helps stimulate interest in the case and makes it more like authentic clinical work. Trigger questions following the case may not have a single correct answer, which allows the group to ponder, collaborate, and practice their clinical reasoning and decision-making skills (Thistlethwaite et al. 2012).

Problem-Based Learning

PBL is a student-centered approach in which small groups of students are presented with trigger materials or real-world clinical problems and work collaboratively to find solutions to problems identified. Small groups (8–10 students) work with a trained facilitator, who guides students to work together to define their learning objectives, ask questions of inquiry, and create and execute a plan using independent research to answer those questions.

Students take on specific roles for each session, including a chair who leads the discussion and keeps the group on track and a scribe who records the discussion and organizes objectives and the identified learning issues. These roles rotate with each case, allowing each member to serve in both roles.

The PBL process involves the following steps for group members, led by the chair and recorded by the scribe:

1. Review the materials recorded by the scribe to identify and clarify unfamiliar terms.
2. Define the problems to be discussed, bringing in a variety of viewpoints on the topic, with problems recorded by the scribe.
3. Brainstorm the problems, allowing members to use previous experience to produce potential explanations and identify areas of incomplete knowledge to research, all recorded by the scribe.
4. Review steps 1–3 to use explanations as tentative solutions, with the scribe reorganizing and restructuring the documentation, if necessary.
5. Formulate learning objectives by group consensus, with the facilitator ensuring that learning objectives are focused, achievable, comprehensive, and appropriate.
6. Study independently to gather information related to learning objectives.
7. In small groups, share the results of independent study, with the facilitator checking learning and potentially assessing the group (Dolmans et al. 2015; Wood 2003).

Benefits and Challenges of CBL and PBL

A key benefit of both CBL and PBL is that they foster a deeper approach to learning than the traditional approach. Students move from reproducing knowledge to application, promoting clinical reasoning, problem-solving, and decision-making skills. By examining real-life, relevant scenarios, students build skills in diagnosis, management, and treatment-planning, which aids their transition to being future providers of patient care. Many students find both approaches more interactive, promoting classroom engagement and solidifying learning. Both modalities allow for the framing of learning from a patient-centered approach. Both are constructivist approaches, built from any existing knowledge students have before the sessions. Finally, the group approach encourages teamwork, problem-solving, and exposure to diverse views (McLean 2016; Thistlethwaite et al. 2012).

Unlike PBL, CBL requires learners to prepare in advance, which needs to be considered in relation to the academic workload; PBL requires no student preparation ahead of time. Both require curriculum and faculty development in the educational modality format. They vary from traditional approaches, requiring faculty to step back from a more traditional "lecture" approach to supporting the group in paving the path toward inquiry. Faculty development may focus more on facilitating and managing group dynamics than giving students answers. CBL benefits from faculty who are also content experts, whereas PBL allows for faculty who may not be specific content experts but still play a pivotal role in keeping the group on task, supported by a facilitator guide that brushes up on specific content expertise.

A challenge with both approaches is that the small group work more intensely uses human resources, requiring faculty members to be present to facilitate all the small groups. In addition, students may not be exposed to the inspirational teachers who traditionally interface with a large group of students. Finally, some students may experience information overload and be unsure of what information is relevant and valuable and how much to study (McLean 2016; Wood 2003).

A Comparison of CBL and PBL

Given the overlap between CBL and PBL, it can be helpful to define the similarities and differences between the two modalities (Table 15.1).

Team-Based Learning

Team-based learning (TBL) is a structured and collaborative learning methodology that helps promote student engagement and accountability for learning (Michaelson and Sweet 2008).

TBL assigns prework before the session and involves a readiness assurance process to assess and incentivize adequate preparation. Thus students come prepared with foundational knowledge, which they use to engage in higher-order learning with their team. These readiness measures are done both individually (individual readiness assessment test [IRAT]) and as a team (group or team readiness assessment test [GRAT or TRAT]), ensuring that each student's foundation and

Table 15.1 Characteristics of CBL and PBL

CBL	Both CBL + PBL	PBL
Has specific learning objectives, with the goal centered around clinical cases, diagnosis, and management Requires advanced study so that learners have base knowledge before class May use more than one case Facilitator is the driver, ensuring learning objectives are met by modeling clinical reasoning	Uses cases in the learning approach, which the facilitator prepares Requires active participation and collaboration of students Builds clinical reasoning skills	Has looser learning objectives, as the process of problem-solving is the focus Does not require advanced study, as learners are expected to research during class Usually uses one case per session Learner is the driver; facilitator role is passive.

Source. McLean 2016; Wood 2003.
Note. CBL = case-based learning; PBL = problem-based learning.

contribution to the group are measured. Once the readiness assessments are concluded, the group facilitator clarifies any misperceptions found in the assessments with a brief didactic session (Burgess et al. 2020; Dolmans et al. 2015; Michaelson and Sweet 2008).

Once the foundation has been established, the group takes on the next step of practicing solving problems, with appropriate problems having real-world relevance and complexity. In the application exercise, students engage in critical thinking, which simulates real-life clinical decision-making. Students practice their communication skills, helping them solidify and develop those skills as part of their professional identity. Given the preparatory work, the team can take on application challenges that are at an increased level of complexity and sophistication and can also use the exercise to work on communication and interpersonal skills.

TBL has many benefits, including the opportunity for students to practice solving real-world problems actively while engaging skills in communication, teamwork, and leadership. The application exercises allow them to engage in deeper learning, and the quizzes and peer evaluation provide real-time feedback so that they can shift their learning and participation strategies if needed. Another benefit is that a large group of students can experience small-group learning with a small number of expert facilitators (Burgess et al. 2020).

TBL requires significant preparation and resource allocation in designing, organizing, and implementing sessions. Tasks include identifying learning outcomes, creating problem-solving activities, writing readiness assurance questions, identifying and potentially developing preparation materials, seeking feedback, and iterating. In addition, time must be allocated to the training of facilitators in the TBL approach to implement a well-organized process that stays on task (Burgess et al. 2020; Michaelson and Sweet 2008).

Simulation-Based Medical Education

Simulation-based medical education (SBME) draws from similar training principles in the aviation industry (another industry that trains individuals to manage high-risk situations in a low-risk and controlled environment). Simulation scenarios bring complexity and authenticity to the replication, giving learners valuable practice time before managing situations in real clinical settings. In addition to mastering technical and nontechnical skills, simulation-based learning also allows students to gain knowledge, mainly through the debriefing and review process; to gain insight into attitudes affecting their development; and to enhance their ability to collaborate in teams. It is immersive, requiring students to engage actively throughout, and performance evaluations can be easily standardized. Learners may practice clinical skills, such as suturing, that require repetition to master (Nestel and Tierney 2007; Piot et al. 2021).

SBME can come in different platforms and is adaptable to many learning objectives. Learners play an active role in the experience, and the simulations should be as accurate to reality as feasible. SBME can use role-play, high-fidelity mannequins, human simulated patients, or even virtual reality. A typical example is mannequins and role-play in basic life support (BLS) training, which is quintessential to mastering this material. Another example is objective structured clinical examinations, in which medical students have short stations to complete during an examination. Each station is typically staffed with simulated patients acting out common presentations, and the students play the role of the physician. Assessments may use direct observation (video recordings), checklist-based evaluations with rating scales, learner-based presentations, or learner-based written exercises (Motola et al. 2013; Piot et al. 2021).

Key features to include as part of SBME are

1. Clear learning objectives
2. Presimulation briefing
3. Simulated scenario in which the students are integral
4. Debriefing

The learning objectives should be clearly defined, and the scenario should suit those objectives. During a presimulation briefing, students should be oriented to the expectations, the learning environment, and any concerns for psychological safety. If video recording or evaluation occurs, students should be properly oriented and give consent. The debrief is best facilitated by someone trained in debriefing, inviting the learners' active involvement. The debrief should address psychological safety relevant to the simulation, such as intense emotional reactions to scenarios and any mistreatment or perceived bias issues. This is an ideal setting for Socratic questioning instead of direct feedback, which can be provided individually to learners if appropriate (Motola et al. 2013).

The benefits of SBME are vast. SBME can be suitable for many types of medical learning requirements, such as repetitive performance (e.g., suturing, history-taking, or physical exams), communication skill-building (e.g., use of empathy or sympathy with simulated patients), team-based skills (e.g., Advanced Cardiac Life Support training), or high-stress or high-stakes performances (e.g., emergency medicine scenarios). SBME promotes person-centered medicine and is a learner-centered educational strategy. Its collaborative nature promotes team training and communication skills. SBME has been shown to improve learning outcomes, enhance patient care and safety, and manage medical errors. Also, it is suitable for many learners because it requires active participation and focuses on reflective understanding and emotional awareness. Simulation is helpful for practice, learning, assessment, and identification of attitudes or biases that may affect the quality of medical care. One key benefit to this modality is the ability for learners to practice and make mistakes without conveying any real risk to patients (Piot et al. 2021).

Standardized evaluations (checklists) and video recording make SBME an excellent means of evaluating and providing meaningful feedback to learners. Not only does it allow individual feedback, but it can also be used to evaluate the strengths and weaknesses of the entire student body. SBME may be integrated with problem-based and case-based models. Also, the advancement of artificial intelligence and virtual reality technology offers opportunities to optimize further simulation-based teaching modalities (Motola et al. 2013).

SBME does come with some challenges. The complexity of the scenarios taught is a primary benefit, but those scenarios are challenging to recreate authentically. Doing so requires that they be broken down into key learning objectives and components. For example, in BLS training, the most critical issues are addressed in simulations, and it is acknowledged that real-life scenarios are less predictable and controlled and come with more nuance. Scenarios involving several roles require finding and training actors capable of appropriately simulating cases, which may be expensive if paid actors are used. This is especially true with more sensitive and specialized roles, such as standardized patients for genital exams. Another challenge with SBME is finding the appropriate setting. One such setting would be mock medical offices equipped with recording equipment. Video recordings may be difficult to set up and expensive and require thoughtful consideration of privacy and consent; however, video recordings can be highly effective for teaching, as students can review their performance and get accurate feedback. A critical consideration in using the SBME format is paying careful attention to maintaining the psychological safety of all participants. As the training is immersive and authentic, learners and facilitators may struggle with difficult emotional experiences. Facilitator development should include how to brief, debrief, and respond to concerns around psychological safety (Motola et al. 2013; Nestel and Tierney 2007; Piot et al. 2021).

Conclusions

Undergraduate medical education has evolved toward highlighting pedagogical approaches that are learner-centered and that allow students to participate actively in building on higher-order thinking skills rather than simply memorizing. These approaches facilitate deeper learning and build critical thinking and teamwork skills, allowing learners to be better prepared for the evolving field of psychiatry. Various approaches have been developed that have shown efficacy in medical education and are helpful in undergraduate psychiatry education. Although these modalities may have some barriers to implementation, learning about them may help leverage the resources necessary to integrate them within an undergraduate psychiatry education curriculum. Doing so allows students to develop their knowledge and skills further, becoming more prepared for the dynamic and complex landscape of psychiatric care ahead of them (Sandrone et al. 2020).

Key Points

- Traditional medical education has relied on passive learning approaches, with teachers delivering content that learners consume. These approaches have significant limitations in preparing future physicians to think critically, keep up with an ever-changing scientific base, and build collaborative skills.
- Several active learning approaches have been developed, including advantages such as critically and deeply examining the material, solving real-world problems, and working collaboratively with peers.

References

Burgess A, van Diggele C, Roberts C, Mellis C: Team-based learning: design, facilitation and participation. BMC Med Educ 20(Suppl 2):461, 2020 33272267

Dolmans D, Michaelsen L, van Merriënboer J, van der Vleuten C: Should we choose between problem-based learning and team-based learning? No, combine the best of both worlds! Med Teach 37(4):354–359, 2015 25154342

Hurtubise L, Hall E, Sheridan L, Han H: The flipped classroom in medical education: engaging students to build competency. J Med Educ Curric Dev 2:JMECD.S23895, 2015

King A: From sage on the stage to guide on the side. Coll Teach 41(1):30–35, 1993

McLean SF: Case-based learning and its application in medical and healthcare fields: a review of worldwide literature. J Med Educ Curric Dev 3:JMECD.S20377, 2016

Michaelsen LK, Sweet M: The essential elements of team-based learning. New Dir Teach Learn 2008(116):7–27, 2008

Motola I, Devine LA, Chung HS, et al: Simulation in healthcare education: a best evidence practical guide. AMEE Guide No. 82. Med Teach 35(10):e1511–e1530, 2013 23941678

Nestel D, Tierney T: Role-play for medical students learning about communication: guidelines for maximising benefits. BMC Med Educ 7(1):3, 2007 17335561

Persky AM, McLaughlin JE: The flipped classroom—from theory to practice in health professional education. Am J Pharm Educ 81(6), 2017

Piot M-A, Attoe C, Billon G, et al: Simulation training in psychiatry for medical education: a review. Front Psychiatry 12:658967, 2021 34093275

Sandrone S, Berthaud JV, Carlson C, et al: Active learning in psychiatry education: current practices and future perspectives. Front Psychiatry 11:211, 2020 32390876

Thistlethwaite JE, Davies D, Ekeocha S, et al: The effectiveness of case-based learning in health professional education: a BEME systematic review: BEME Guide No. 23. Med Teach 34(6):e421–e444, 2012 22578051

Wood DF: Problem based learning. BMJ 326(7384):328–330, 2003 12574050

16

Remote Learning and New Technologies in the Teaching of Psychiatry

John Luo, M.D.
Kalyn Reddy, M.D., M.P.H.

Undergraduate medical education has been at the forefront of innovation by implementing technology to engage learners and enhance retention of the material. Medical students at many institutions have access to recorded lectures in case of absence and to serve as a reference for later review. They often take advantage of these recordings by reviewing them during mandatory attendance lectures, which enables them to accomplish more in the time allocated for studying. Many students even watch the recordings at double speed to increase efficiency.

The technology used in undergraduate medical education is not just for the convenience of students and faculty, however. The Liaison Committee on Medical Education (LCME), the accrediting body for medical education programs leading to a medical doctor degree, has created principles that medical schools must follow to maintain accreditation while using spatial or temporal learning (LCME 2015). No matter how the medical school delivers educational content, LCME expects that the school will comply with all standards and demonstrate satisfactory performance with all elements for accreditation.

Characteristics of New Learners

People of any age will have their expectations and worldview affected by significant events during their formative years; such events are called period effects (Williams et al. 2017). The most recent and widely experienced period effect was the global COVID-19 pandemic, which involved a sudden shift to fully remote learning and work. Most medical students in the coming years were in school during the pandemic and experienced at least some fully remote learning before matriculation in medical school. Individual preferences will vary, but we predict widespread familiarity and comfort with virtual learning as the norm for current and future students.

The span of any generation's birth years can vary by source. According to the Pew Research Center, Millennials were born from 1981 to 1996, and members of Generation Z (Gen Z) were born starting in 1997 (Dimock 2019). Here we explore generational trends, focusing on Gen Z students (who will make up most medical school classes in the coming years). The trends relating to technology are broadly applicable to Millennials, too, and where pertinent differences exist, we note them (Williams et al. 2017). Although these trends will not apply to every person who falls within the described age ranges and should not be overly generalized, they can help bridge communication and are one tool to examine how to best structure undergraduate medical education (Williams et al. 2017). Further, medical students are a self-selected and academically selected group and may systematically differ in some ways from their broader age cohort.

Gen Z is often regarded as the "digital natives," and many monikers center around their use of technology and the internet (Kirschner and De Bruyckere 2017; Prensky 2001). They tend toward high usage of smart devices, are generally comfortable with virtual meetings, and have a pronounced preference for electronic learning materials, exams, and communication methods (Plochocki 2019; Talmon 2019). A Gen Z individual consumes about 9 hours of digital content and 70 videos daily (Talmon 2019). Many use YouTube to learn and as a platform for observing experts performing tasks (Seemiller and Grace 2017). Many also create content, especially on social media platforms such as TikTok (Talmon 2019).

Gen Z students' familiarity with user reviews and digital interactions fosters an expectation for real-time feedback (Talmon 2019) (see later section, "Polling"). Compared with Millennials, they may prefer structured activities and guidance rather than open-ended tasks, and they have a greater tendency toward individual rather than collaborative learning (Plochocki 2019; Seemiller and Grace 2017). Social influence plays a vital role in how members of Gen Z adopt technology (Aydin 2022). Though they are often regarded as native technology users, it is wrong to assume technological literacy or a greater ability to learn new information (Kennedy and Fox 2013; Kirschner and De Bruyckere 2017). They may have a preference for "bite-sized" content and a greater tendency to switch between tasks frequently (Talmon 2019). This should not be mistaken for multitasking (the ability to do several things simultaneously) or conflated with greater efficiency in learning and understanding material (Kirschner and De Bruyckere 2017). Distinguishing fact and opinion may be more difficult for Gen Z students, who may struggle to connect ideas (Talmon 2019). Educators should not assume that high internet use translates to an intrinsic ability to find and accurately apply scientific knowledge. Scientific literacy remains an imperative element of medical education.

Advantages of Remote Learning

Video conferencing offers many obvious advantages for remote learners and educators alike. Travel, parking, and having to locate an unfamiliar classroom or lecture hall are eliminated. Busy educators can fit in more lectures and meetings in a day without having to account for time spent in transit; likewise, medical students at different and distant clinical sites can do more clinical work without allowing time to travel. Faculty or students who attending conferences in another city and time zone can still attend educational sessions without missing any valuable content or declining their assigned teaching session. The COVID-19 pandemic highlighted how grand rounds speakers from external organizations who could not travel could still contribute to the educational mission, and these speakers could fit more engagements in their schedule without the travel time and cost. Many organizations discovered that attendance at grand rounds for faculty, resident physicians, and medical students reached historic levels, given the ease of attendance.

The pandemic accelerated the development and deployment of remote learning out of sheer necessity, when medical students had to stay home as a precaution. Smith and Boscak (2021) described success in pivoting from on-site clinical radiology rotations to self-study educational resources, independent review of unknown cases using a virtual workstation, and online interactive conferences. Postcourse surveys revealed that students strongly agreed that the course was clinically relevant, with accessible and engaging material, as it implemented flipped-classroom techniques that incorporated independent individual learning with subsequent instructor-led interactive sessions. Stock and Singh (2023) used Google Forms to create patient case scenarios with multiple-choice questions based on learning objectives and framed in a clinical context. They used an "escape room" format that required a mastery of concepts to progress through the cases. Analytics from surveys at the end of the exercises showed that 94% of students found it an effective learning tool that was easy to navigate and recommended it for use in future courses.

Remote learning showcases its main strength when a specialized curriculum can be shared with multiple institutions and collaborators. For example, the National Curriculum in Reproductive Psychiatry (https://ncrptraining.org/about/) answers a shortage of faculty to teach reproductive psychiatry at residency programs, as the Accreditation Council for Graduate Medical Education (ACGME) does not require reproductive psychiatry. The curriculum provides reproductive psychiatry materials developed by national experts to be used in the classroom by nonexpert facilitators, who volunteer their time to contribute to accessing the curriculum. Similarly, the Providers Clinical Support System-Medications for Opioid Use Disorders (PCSS-MOUD) (https://pcssnow.org/about/), funded by the Substance Abuse and Mental Health Services Administration (SAMHSA), provides evidence-based practices to improve health care and outcomes those at risk for substance use disorders and treatment for individuals with opioid use disorder. PCSS-MOUD has collaborated with the African American Behavioral Health Center of Excellence (https://africanamericanbehavioralhealth.org/about/about-us.aspx) to address the urgent need for more significant equity and effectiveness in behavioral health services for African Americans. These are just a few examples of how remote learning transcends time and distance to make expertise widely available.

Gamification in Medical Education

Gamification is the term used for including game attributes in nongaming contexts such as education. An early and popular tool is Kahoot! (https://kahoot.com), which helps create assessment tools in the form of quiz games. Students see a question in the classroom and answer on their phones. Points are assigned for both speed and accuracy. Learners are engaged through the use of whimsical music and graphics and the competitive race to answer the fastest. There are additional tools, such as word clouds, picture reveals, and an updated leaderboard after each question. The main caveat when using Kahoot! is that the presenter and attendees must have wireless internet access. One alternative is to use Microsoft PowerPoint for a Jeopardy!-style game (Lloyd 2025)—scores are not graded automatically, and the instructor must choose whoever raises their hand first in the classroom or video conference.

Van Gaalen et al. (2021), in their systematic review on the effectiveness of gamification approaches in education for the health professions, found that there was increased use of the learning material with some improved learning outcomes. Notably, they identified no adverse outcomes in the papers that met their review criteria. Gamified training helps engage medical students with a high degree of technological literacy who desire an interactive educational experience (Krishnamurthy et al. 2022). Game-based learning adds diverse game elements to encourage engagement and raise participants' enthusiasm (Xu 2023). Other potential advantages of gamified training platforms include enhanced collaboration, real-world application, clinical decision-making, distance training, learning analytics, and swift feedback (McCoy et al. 2016). There is good evidence that serious gaming was at least as effective as traditional learning regarding knowledge and skills (Gentry et al. 2019).

An example of serious gaming for health education is Septris (https://med.stanford.edu/septris.html). This online educational game was developed to teach hospital-based medical, surgical, intensive care, and emergency department physicians and nurses to treat sepsis. The game's goal is to heal 10 patients. Clicking on a patient portrait shows vitals, history, and lab results. Selecting tests, administering intravenous fluids, and ordering consultations from the ICU are ways to treat the patient. Ultimately, the patient will either be healed or die based on players' decisions. This learning module offers continuing medical and nursing education credits.

Polls

The use of interactive polling has shifted learning from passive to active (Brezis and Cohen 2004), with engagement found in Kahoot!- and Jeopardy!-style presentations. Gone are the expensive and cumbersome audience response systems that required a receiver and multiple transmitters for each audience member and software on a computer to display the responses by percentages. Those earlier systems were also quite limited regarding question type and fixed responses. Now, with web-based online systems (see Table 16.1), all you need is internet access on the computer with the presentation and participants who use a mobile phone, tablet, or computer. Audience response has expanded beyond multiple-choice questions to include word clouds, open-ended text responses, ranking choices, rating scales, and XY plots. Depending on the vendor, there may be integration within PowerPoint, Prezi, Google Slides, or Keynote presentation software. As with any presentation feature, judicious use of polls and other interactive elements is critical to maintaining audience interest and engagement.

Podcasts

In recent years, podcasts have emerged as a powerful tool in medical education. Originally a portmanteau of "iPod" and "broadcast," podcasts are digital audio files (and occasionally videos) available for streaming or download onto a computer, tablet, or smartphone (Newman et al. 2021; Shapiro 2022).

Podcasts offer numerous advantages as an educational tool—mainly cost-effectiveness, flexibility, and ease of use (Newman et al. 2021). They can be easily stored on mobile devices, facilitating learning on-the-go—a boon for busy medical students who can listen while exercising, commuting to clinic sites, or traveling to campus. Moreover,

Table 16.1 Online Polling Sites

Polleverywhere.com
SurveyMonkey.com
Mentimeter.com
Slido.com
Doodle.com
Easypolls.net
Directpoll.com
Vevox.com

the downloadable nature of podcasts allows for uninterrupted learning in areas with limited internet access. The on-demand feature of podcasts empowers learners to steer their learning path by selecting topics that pique their interest and are relevant to their stage of training. It also allows them to learn at times that work with their schedules (Rodman and Trivedi 2020).

Myriad podcasts are targeted for teaching medical students. Some are specific to psychiatry, and others are more general, targeted at preparing students for U.S. Medical Licensing Exams (USMLE) (too many to name) or clerkships (Bradford 2018). Still others focus on career preparation, offering information on various specialties (Drummond 2016–2019) and applying to residencies. Some examples of psychiatry-specific podcasts that may be appropriate for medical students include: PsychEd (2017–2025), Psychiatry Boot Camp (Mullen 2023–2025), Psychiatry Explored (2021–2025), and the Carlat Psychiatry Podcast (Newsome and Aiken 2023–2025).

Clinical educators can also create their own podcasts if they wish. Doing so is a fresh way of reaching students that also allows reaching learners outside of their institution. Relevant considerations for the educator who ventures into podcasting include determining the podcast length, securing a host, finding a suitable hosting platform, ensuring high audio quality with appropriate equipment and sound engineering team, and securing the necessary funding (Newman et al. 2021). Setting up a podcast can be quite budget-friendly, as demonstrated by an emergency medicine student interest group at Oregon Health and Science University, which initiated a podcast with a budget of $400 (Lichtenheld et al. 2015). Institutions can incentivize and support content creation by considering podcasts part of academic portfolios for faculty promotion and tenure (Cabrera et al. 2017).

There are some potential concerns and pitfalls when using podcasts in medical education. Typically, podcasts are organized chronologically, making it difficult to locate topic-specific content (Rodman and Trivedi 2020). Students may find different podcast series relevant at various points of their education, partially mitigating this issue. The podcast most appropriate as they prepare for Step 1 is likely not the same one they will listen to during their psychiatry subinternship. Additionally, the lack of a standardized vetting or peer-review process raises concerns over accuracy and relevance of the content, primarily when sourced outside the institution (Rodman and Trivedi 2020). Thus, fostering students' academic and technological literacy is essential for effectively using this valuable platform (Lichtenheld et al. 2015).

Flipped Classroom

Technology can be an important aid for active learning. As discussed in Chapter 15, "Beyond Lecturing," active learning approaches such as flipped classrooms require preparatory materials so that the learner is prepared to use interactive sessions to apply knowledge gained during preparation. Preparatory materials include videos, primary research, podcasts, educational games, quizzes, and interactive online tools. Content can be created specifically for the curriculum or drawn from outside sources. Assigned materials should not be too time-intensive or excessively detailed for the level of the learner. For example, assigning a textbook as preparation for a workshop or series of workshops is unrealistic. The assigned materials should be comprehensive enough that students grasp the necessary material to prepare for the session but not so detailed that they cannot complete them or that the session becomes redundant (Ramnanan and Pound 2017).

Based on the current literature, our recommendation is strongest for preparatory work to take the form of video content, ideally created explicitly for your flipped classroom curriculum. Students engage more with video content than other preparatory materials and report being more likely to prepare for flipped classroom sessions when given videos rather than reading materials (Bordes et al. 2021; Ramnanan and Pound 2017; Smith and Boscak 2021). This gravitation toward video content aligns with the preferences of current learners described earlier. Video content is most effective and well received when regularly integrated as part of the curriculum and created explicitly for the flipped classroom model (as opposed to providing video recordings of previously recorded lectures) (Bordes et al. 2021). The optimal length of a video will vary depending on the content, but consider providing videos shorter than the traditional 50–90-minute lecture. Approximately 20 minutes is a reasonable maximum length for educational videos (Bordes et al. 2021; Hew and Lo 2018). More research is needed on incorporating videos into medical education (Hew and Lo 2018). This is a rapidly changing area of technology, and options and recommendations for creating and distributing educational video content to learners will continue to evolve.

With recorded video (as opposed to live in-person or video lectures), learners can watch the video several times, pause to look things up, and speed up or slow down the lecture speed to their preference (Hew and Lo 2018). Students can consume recorded materials at their own time and pace, allowing greater flexibility and autonomy over their learning. Educators likewise can record educational content entirely asynchronously (for example, on their administrative days or during lighter workweeks) to be viewed later by students at their convenience. The administrative burden is reduced, as coordinators are freed from juggling the schedules of various lecturers. Prerecorded lectures can be made from any location, decreasing the educational barrier for off-site experts or educators from other institutions (Grant et al. 2021). Efficiency is improved by eliminating travel time and creating educational material that is easy to distribute widely. Recorded content can be created with specialty software (e.g., Panopto, Camtasia), Zoom recordings, or YouTube.

Consider starting flipped classroom sessions with a brief quiz on the assigned material (Hew and Lo 2018). Quizzes reinforce the material, may help students recall the information they learned during independent study, help instructors gauge understanding of the material, identify areas that need clarification or review, and can act as a gentle motivator to complete the presession assignments (Hailikari et al. 2008; Hew and Lo 2018) (also see earlier section, "Polling").

Anki

Anki is a free-to-use, open-source flashcard program that helps with spaced repetition learning. Students can create their own cards with information they are attempting to master, such as the types of personality disorders or their definitions (Anki 2023). Anki cards can include images. Users can synchronize the cards across multiple devices with an account on https://ankiweb.net and share their decks with others. Students who use Anki have demonstrated higher USMLE Step I scores (Lu et al. 2021). A recent cohort study assessing the impact of Anki use among medical students at Boonshoft School of Medicine showed that Anki users scored significantly higher on the course exams and the Comprehensive Basic Science Exam (Gilbert et al. 2023). Anki has become very popular among medical students as a tool to help them learn, partly because they learn what content is important and create their flashcards accordingly, helping them to review and synthesize their knowledge.

Artificial Intelligence

Artificial or augmented intelligence (AI) use has been innovative but controversial in recent years. It provides an opportunity for creativity in medical education but can also invoke fears related to job insecurity and being replaced by computers. Torous and Greenberg (2025), in a 2025 editorial in *Academic Psychiatry*, concluded that AI and large language models in psychiatry medical education can augment but will not replace current best practices. There are many potential uses of artificial intelligence in undergraduate medical education, and some medical educators have already begun integrating AI. Harvard Medical School is building artificial intelligence into the curriculum to help train medical students (Gehrman 2024). In the health sciences and technology track, a month-long course will cover the limitations of AI use in clinical decision-making and machine-learning skills. In an American Medical Association interview, associate dean of medical informatics and director of the Institute for Innovations in Medical Education at the New York University Grossman School of Medicine in New York, Dr. Marc Triola, described a project called DX Mentor, with which NYU uses AI to automatically identify just-in-time learning resources and medical literature based on the diagnoses of the patients that medical students are caring for (Unger 2024).

Potential applications of AI for the psychiatry educator are numerous. In a scoping review of generative AI in psychiatric education, Lee et al. (2025) identified almost 13,000 papers about using AI in case-based learning, simulation, content synthesis, and assessment. Smith et al. (2023) used ChatGPT version 3.5 to aid in the teaching of social psychiatry and prompted it to write a fictionalized case vignette regarding a migrant who recently moved to a new country and experienced mental health issues. Versus a clinician-generated vignette, the AI-generated vignette included a greater variety of psychopathological symptoms that could be used to teach differential diagnoses and stimulate discussion regarding the treatment plan and social determinants of health. Hudon et al. (2024) described how they used ChatGPT in psychiatry to develop script concordance tests in undergraduate medical education. Clinical scenarios with multiple-choice and open-ended questions generated by ChatGPT and expert clinicians were compared: test takers could not distinguish which were written by ChatGPT and which were written by experts. The key for psychiatric educators in deciding how to implement AI technology in undergraduate medical education is understanding how the models work. One of the major components is Bayesian statistics, which looks at prior beliefs and updates them as new data are available (Soriano 2024).

A series of coin flips can be an illustrative example. A coin flipped repeatedly should result in a 50–50 distribution of head versus tails over time. This is our prior probability, our initial expectation of what outcome is likely to occur. However, if the coin reaches heads 70 out of 100 flips, this pattern now indicates that the likelihood is that the coin is imbalanced in some way. We can use these data to update our expectations and obtain a new (posterior) probability that the coin will land on heads. The posterior probability is that the coin will deliver heads 70% of the time in the future. AI systems similarly adjust as they receive and incorporate new information. Stryker and Holdsworth (2024) explained that natural language processing enables computers to understand and communicate with human language by combining computational linguistics with machine learning. Kapronczay and Urwin (2025), in their introduction to large language models (LLMs), clarified that these models use machine learning to conduct a probability distribution over words or word sequences. These LLMs learn from human-generated text sources such as Wikipedia, textbooks, newspapers, and transcripts of telephone conversations. When a user enters a prompt, otherwise known as a query or input, into an LLM, the program generates a response based on the probability that the generated text is the answer to the query. Such data processing requires high processing power, which is why artificial intelligence has recently become more widespread.

It is crucial to understand the limitations of LLMs. An LLM is a predictive engine that pulls patterns together based on its training text and produces more text based on patterns and probability. It does not have any understanding of language, math, or facts. For this reason, it can *hallucinate*, or generate an output that is not real (Neto 2023). AI models are often termed *black boxes*, providing outputs for which the decision-making process is unclear (Carabantes 2020). This lack of transparency is particularly problematic for educational settings in which learners aim to develop diagnostic and treatment-planning skills. Models also may have *bias and discrimination* from either the original training data or the AI algorithm (Holdsworth 2023). *Privacy* is another concern, especially with the use of publicly accessible LLMs. Any data uploaded into the LLM can be retained as learning material, so any protected health information, as outlined in the Health Insurance Portability and Accountability Act of 1996 (Pub. L. No. 104-191), must be used in a secured setting with a business associate contract. With such power of AI technology to predict suicide risk or make psychiatric diagnoses, there are ethical concerns regarding appropriate use. Issues related to justice, health equity, algorithmic bias, discrimination based on demographic characteristics, preservation of patient autonomy and privacy, trust in the health care system, and beneficence must all be considered. Ethical guidelines related to AI have been and will continue to be developed by governments and medical organizations (American Medical Association 2023; Kumari et al. 2025).

Artificial intelligence offers transformative potential for undergraduate medical education in psychiatry, addressing longstanding challenges while creating new opportunities to enhance learning. As these technologies evolve, their thoughtful integration—guided by educational principles, ethical considerations, and ongoing evaluation—will be essential to preparing the next generation of physicians to provide compassionate, evidence-based psychiatric care.

Faculty Development

Faculty development may be necessary to help faculty implement remote learning and innovative technologies in medical education. Depending on their technical skill, some innovations, such as podcasts, sound easy enough, but there is a learning curve regarding editing and incorporating transitions. The resources required for the quality of the audio and video desired may be beyond the budget of the faculty member. Many medical schools have information technology support teams to help faculty create content, but the focus has also shifted to adding students as content creators. The iMedEd Initiative at the University of California Irvine School of Medicine (https://imeded.uci.edu) will provide every student arriving in 2026 with an iPad and a handheld ultrasound device, with the goal that students curate and create content, including AnkiMobile flashcards, as well as clinically correlate findings with their ultrasound machines. Not all technology is challenging, since Kahoot! is easy to create and implement. Much will depend on the faculty member's time and desire to learn new technologies from medical students who are digital natives.

Conclusions

Remote learning and new innovative technologies have helped medical schools meet the needs of their learners whose learning preferences have changed from traditional lecture-only didactics to more interactive learning. Strategies range from simple to complex, using video conferencing (both live and recorded), creating podcasts and flashcards, mixing in polling for interaction, and creating a competitive game environment to increase engagement and retention of materials. Virtual and augmented reality are beginning to be incorporated into education (Miltykh et al. 2023). Most would agree that the COVID-19 pandemic was not a positive experience, but it certainly was a catalyst for remote learning and innovative technology adoption in medical education. These technologies and innovations bridge the gaps regarding the learning preferences of millennials and Gen Z, the distance between faculty and students, the need to travel, and the timing of events. Medical schools are often at the forefront of implementing these technologies to meet the needs of medical students, but having such technologies helps with recruitment as well. Likewise, medical students are increasingly becoming content creators and innovators. Medical education will continue to evolve with the new technologies and strategies.

Key Points

- New learners are comfortable with new technologies and have a distinct preference for using them.
- Remote learning bridges the difference in time zones, locations, and travel demands.
- Remote learning also creates a need to implement new technologies and strategies such as gaming, polling, or flipped-classroom techniques to achieve high levels of engagement.
- Recorded content (such as podcasts and lectures) provides opportunities for on-demand learning that the new generation prefers.

References

American Medical Association: AMA issues new principles for AI development, deployment and use. American Medical Association, 2023. Available at: https://www.ama-assn.org/press-center/press-releases/ama-issues-new-principles-ai-development-deployment-use. Accessed April 11, 2025.

Anki. Application. Available at: https://apps.ankiweb.net. Accessed September 28, 2023.

Aydin G, Kumru S: Paving the way for increased e-health record use: elaborating intentions of Gen-Z. Health Syst (Basingstoke) 12(3):281–298, 2022

Bordes SJ, Walker D, Modica LJ, et al: Towards the optimal use of video recordings to support the flipped classroom in medical school basic sciences education. Med Educ Online 26(1):1841406, 2021 33119431

Bradford J: Medical Student StudyCast, 2018. Podcast.

Brezis M, Cohen R: Interactive learning in medicine: Socrates in electronic clothes. QJM 97(1):47–51, 2004 14702511

Cabrera D, Vartabedian BS, Spinner RJ, et al: More than likes and tweets: creating social media portfolios for academic promotion and tenure. J Grad Med Educ 9(4):421–425, 2017 28824752

Carabantes M: Black-box artificial intelligence: an epistemological and critical analysis. AI Soc 35(2):309–317, 2020

Dimock M: Defining Generations: Where Millennials End and Generation Z Begins. Pew Research Center (blog), 2019. Available at: https://www.pewresearch.org/short-reads/2019/01/17/where-millennials-end-and-generation-z-begins/. Accessed September 22, 2023.

Drummond I: The Undifferentiated Medical Student, 2016–2019. Podcast. Available at: https://www.undifferentiatedmedicalstudent.com/. Accessed June 24, 2025.

Gehrman E: How Generative AI Is Transforming Medical Education. Harvard Medicine Magazine, 2024. Available at: https://magazine.hms.harvard.edu/articles/how-generative-ai-transforming-medical-education. Accessed April 10, 2025.

Gentry SV, Gauthier A, L'Estrade Ehrstrom B, et al: Serious gaming and gamification education in health professions: systematic review. J Med Internet Res 28;21(3):e12994, 2019 30920375

Gilbert MM, Frommeyer TC, Brittain GV, et al: A cohort study assessing the impact of Anki as a spaced repetition tool on academic performance in medical school. Med Sci Educ 33(4):955–962, 2023 37546209

Grant LL, Opperman MJ, Schiller B, et al: Medical student engagement in a virtual learning environment positively correlates with course performance and satisfaction in psychiatry. Med Sci Educ 31(3):1133–1140, 2021 33868773

Hailikari T, Katajavuori N, Lindblom-Ylanne S: The relevance of prior knowledge in learning and instructional design. Am J Pharm Educ 72(5):113, 2008 19214267

Hew KF, Lo CK: Flipped classroom improves student learning in health professions education: a meta-analysis. BMC Med Educ 18(1):38, 2018 29544495

Holdsworth J: What Is AI Bias? IBM, 2023. Available at: https://www.ibm.com/think/topics/ai-bias. Accessed April 11, 2025.

Hudon A, Kiepura B, Pelletier M, Phan V: Using ChatGPT in psychiatry to design script concordance tests in undergraduate medical education: mixed methods study. JMIR Med Educ 10:e54067, 2024 38596832

Kapronczay M, Urwin M: A Beginner's Guide to Language Models. Built In, 2025. Available at: https://builtin.com/data-science/beginners-guide-language-models. Accessed April 11, 2025.

Kennedy DM, Fox R: 'Digital natives': an Asian perspective for using learning technologies. Int J Educ Dev Using ICT 9(1):65–79, 2013

Kirschner PA, De Bruyckere P: The myths of the digital native and the multitasker. Teach Teach Educ 67(October):135–142, 2017

Krishnamurthy K, Selvaraj N, Gupta P, et al: Benefits of gamification in medical education. Clin Anat 35(6):795–807, 2022 35637557

Kumari R, Das S, Singh RK: Ethical Considerations in AI Powered Diagnosis and Treatment, in Responsible and Explainable Artificial Intelligence in Healthcare. Edited by Singh A, Singh KK, Izonin I. New York, Academic Press, 2025, pp 25–53

Lee QY, Chen M, Ong CW, Ho CSH: The role of generative artificial intelligence in psychiatric education—a scoping review. BMC Med Educ 25(1):438, 2025 40133891

Liaison Committee on Medical Education: Accreditation Issues Related to Spatial and Temporal Distance Learning. LCME, 2015. Available at: https://lcme.org/wp-content/uploads/2025/04/Accreditation-Issues_Spatial-and-Temporal-Distance-Learning_2025-04-10.docx. Accessed June 24, 2023.

Lichtenheld A, Nomura M, Chapin N, et al: Development and implementation of an emergency medicine podcast for medical students: EMIGcast. West J Emerg Med 16(6):877–878, 2015 26594282

Lloyd J: How to Make a Jeopardy Game on PowerPoint. wikiHow, 2025. Available at: https://www.wikihow.com/Make-a-Jeopardy-Game-on-PowerPoint. Accessed June 24, 2025.

Lu M, Farhat JH, Beck Dallaghan GL: Enhanced learning and retention of medical knowledge using the mobile flash card application Anki. Med Sci Educ 31(6):1975–1981, 2021 34956708

McCoy L, Lewis JH, Dalton D: Gamification and multimedia for medical education: a landscape review. J Am Osteopath Assoc 116(1):22–34, 2016 26745561

Miltykh I, Kafarov ES, Covantsev S, et al: A new dimension in medical education: virtual reality in anatomy during COVID-19 pandemic. Clin Anat 36(7):1007–1015, 2023 37485993

Mullen M: Psychiatry Boot Camp, 2023–2025. Podcast. Available at: https://podcasts.apple.com/us/podcast/psychiatry-boot-camp/id1671902940. Accessed June 24, 2025.

Neto JAR. Chat GPT and the Generative AI Hallucinations. Medium, 2023. Available at: https://medium.com/chatgpt-learning/chatgtp-and-the-generative-ai-hallucinations-62feddc72369. Accessed April 11, 2025.

Newsome K, Aiken C: The Carlat Psychiatry Podcast, 2023–2025. Podcast. Available at: https://www.thecarlatreport.com/blogs/2-the-carlat-psychiatry-podcast. Accessed June 24, 2025.

Newman J, Liew A, Bowles J, et al: Podcasts for the delivery of medical education and remote learning. J Med Internet Res 27;23(8):e29168, 2021 34448719

Plochocki JH: Several ways generation Z may shape the medical school landscape. J Med Educ Curric Dev 6(January):2382120519884325, 2019 31701014

Prensky M: Digital natives, digital immigrants part 2: do they really think differently? On the Horizon 9(6):1–6, 2001

PsychEd, 2017–2025. Podcast. Available at: https://www.psychedpodcast.org/. Accessed June 24, 2025.

Psychiatry Explored, 2021–2025. Podcast. Available at: https://podcasts.apple.com/us/podcast/psychiatry-explored/id1601123546. Accessed June 24, 2025.

Ramnanan CJ, Pound LD: Advances in medical education and practice: student perceptions of the flipped classroom. Adv Med Educ Pract 8(January):63–73, 2017 28144171

Rodman A, Trivedi S: Podcasting: a roadmap to the future of medical education. Semin Nephrol 40(3):279–283, 2020 32560776

Seemiller C, Grace M: Generation Z: educating and engaging the next generation of students. About Campus 22(3):21–26, 2017

Shapiro A: The iPod is dead, but the podcast lives on. 2022. Available at: https://www.theverge.com/2022/5/15/23071515/ipod-dead-podcast-legacy-apple-spotify. Accessed June 5, 2024.

Smith E, Boscak A: A virtual emergency: learning lessons from remote medical student education during the COVID-19 pandemic. Emerg Radiol 28(3):445–452, 2021 33420528

Smith A, Hachen S, Schleifer R, et al: Old dog, new tricks? Exploring the potential functionalities of ChatGPT in supporting educational methods in social psychiatry. Int J Soc Psychiatry 69(8):1882–1889, 2023 37392000

Soriano J: What Is Bayesian Statistics? A Complete Guide for Beginners. Quant Matter, 2024. Available at: https://quantmatter.com/what-is-bayesian-statistics-a-complete-guide-for-beginners/. Accessed April 11, 2025.

Stock A, Singh P: Online medical education: utilization of Google Forms for remote active learning experiences in a large medical school class during the COVID-19 pandemic. Med Sci Educ 33(2):333–335, 2023 36811081

Stryker C, Holdsworth J. What Is Natural Language Processing? IBM, 2024. Available at: https://www.ibm.com/think/topics/natural-language-processing. Accessed April 11, 2025.

Talmon GA: Generation Z: what's next? Med Sci Educ 29(1)(Suppl 1):9–11, 2019 34457613

Torous J, Greenberg W: Large language models and artificial intelligence in psychiatry medical education: augmenting but not replacing best practices. Acad Psychiatry 49(1):22–24, 2025 39107543

Unger T: ChatGPT in medical education: generative AI and the future of artificial intelligence in health care. AMA Digital Health, 2024. Available at: https://www.ama-assn.org/practice-management/digital/chatgpt-medical-education-generative-ai-and-future-artificial. Accessed April 10, 2025.

van Gaalen AEJ, Brouwer J, Schönrock-Adema J, et al: Gamification of health professions education: a systematic review. Adv Health Sci Educ Theory Pract 26(2):683–711, 2021 33128662

Williams VN, Medina J, Medina A, et al: Bridging the millennial generation expectation gap: perspectives and strategies for physician and interprofessional faculty. Am J Med Sci 353(2):109–115, 2017

Xu M, Luo Y, Zhang Y, et al: Game-based learning in medical education. Front Public Health 11:1113682, 2023

17

The Role of Simulation in Teaching Psychiatry to Medical Students[1]

Helen L. Dainton-Howard, M.D.
Christine M. Pelic, M.D.
Andrew R. Alkis, M.D.
Christopher G. Pelic, M.D.

Traditional medical education is rooted in the nineteenth-century ideology pioneered by Sir William Osler that students should learn medicine through direct patient experiences, complemented by classroom learning (McGaghie 2015). Throughout the twentieth century, there was growing concern that undergraduate medical education placed too high an emphasis on scientific knowledge and not enough on critical thinking, decision-making, procedural skills, and compassionate, empathetic listening (Campbell et al. 2023; Cooke et al. 2006). Encouraged by

[1] This chapter is adapted from McGue SR, Pelic CM, McCadden A, et al: The use of simulation in teaching. Psychiatr Clin 44(2):159–171, 2021. Used with permission. Copyright © Elsevier 2021.

the Accreditation Council for Graduate Medical Education (ACGME), medical schools began placing a greater focus on experiential learning modalities that can offer students an environment to learn, engage more directly in realistic problem-solving, and allow a supportive environment to learn from their experience (Campbell et al. 2023; Wijnen-Meijer et al. 2013). Simulation-based medical education (SBME) has been one answer to this call (Campbell et al. 2023; Cooke et al. 2006).

Simulation is defined by David Gaba as "a technique, not a technology, to replace or amplify real experiences with guided experiences that evoke or replicate substantial aspects of the real world in a fully interactive manner" (Gaba 2004, p. i2; Herrera-Aliaga and Estrada 2022). Simulation allows for the standardization of educational experiences, which is hard to achieve in clinical settings. In addition, simulating high-risk scenarios in a safe environment can help efficiently teach crisis management skills (Armenia et al. 2018; Institute of Medicine Committee on Quality of Health Care 2000) without putting patients at risk during the learning process. Simulation also allows for quality improvement, error reduction, communication skills improvement, and most importantly, patient safety. Because of these advantages, SBME has been widely adopted in undergraduate and graduate programs (Passiment et al. 2011). According to the Association of American Medical Colleges (AAMC) (2011), simulation is arguably the most prominent innovation in medical education in recent history.

SBME is especially helpful in psychiatric education because direct observation of patient care and immediate feedback to the trainee can be difficult to achieve. Observing residents as they build rapport with the patients in their clinic panel, for example, could violate the privacy required for developing a psychiatrist–patient relationship and diminish trust by potentially conveying that teaching is prioritized over patient care (Beutler and Harwood 2004). There is also significant heterogeneity in psychiatry, making uniformity in clinical experience challenging for clerkship directors to provide to medical students.

Selecting a simulation modality most often depends on the educational goals of the activity and the resources available. Modalities exist on a wide spectrum, distinguished by fidelity (level of realism), technology, and required instructor/operator expertise (Herrera-Aliaga and Estrada 2022). Simulation modalities can be classified into six major groups (Beutler and Harwood 2004; Ziv et al. 2000, 2003):

1. Low-technology: low-cost models or mannequins used to teach basic knowledge or psychomotor skills

2. Simulated/standardized patients (SPs): actors trained to portray patients who can facilitate teaching and assessment of history-taking, physical examination, communication skills, and professionalism
3. Screen-based computer simulators: software for training and assessment of clinical knowledge and decision-making that may include artificial intelligence (AI)
4. Complex task trainers: computer-based programs for high-fidelity procedural skills
5. High-fidelity patient simulators: computer-based mannequins replicating complex and high-risk clinical conditions in lifelike settings
6. Virtual reality: emerging technology that involves sensory inputs and various user receptors (e.g., head tracker); may be used for various learning and assessment purposes

Evidence has shown that simulation benefits educational outcomes (Cook et al. 2013; McGaghie et al. 2014; Sperling et al. 2013). Areas that warrant further research include the impact on patient outcomes, sustainability of simulation efforts, and cost-effectiveness of training programs (Armenia et al. 2018).

Demonstrating the effectiveness of simulation is important because there are significant costs associated with implementing and maintaining simulation in medical curricula. Purchasing and maintaining equipment, university space, and faculty hours in curriculum development and implementation are all costs that must be considered for each institution (Lentz et al. 2005). Evidence for effectiveness can also help overcome educational inertia, which is described as the interacting factors that lead medical schools to resist change in education (Jónasson 2016; McGaghie 2015).

History of Simulation-Based Medical Education

Simulation was adopted in other fields before the recent medical education boom. Simulation is critical in high-risk sectors where the consequence of human error can be dire. Unsurprisingly, simulation first became widespread in aviation, aeronautics, and nuclear safety. The military has long used simulation as a mode of preparation and training—the modern military accounted for 80% of all modeling and simulation work before the 1990s (Rosen 2008). It is also not surprising that in health care, emergency medicine and critical care were the first to broadly incorporate simulation into medical education (Piot et al. 2021).

There are examples of simulation in medical education throughout history. Models have long been used to help students learn about anatomical structures. In China in 1027 AD, the imperial physician Wang Wei-Yi had two life-size bronze statues made for teaching surface anatomy and location of acupuncture points (Owen 2012; Schnorrenberger 2008). In the eighteenth century, two surgeons working separately in Bologna and Paris developed birthing simulator models to teach delivery techniques to address high infant and maternal mortality rates (Buck 1991; Jones et al. 2015; Owen 2012; Rosen 2008). The early twentieth century saw the arrival of "Ms. Chase," a full-body simulator developed by Hartford Hospital to assist nursing students in training (Herrera-Aliaga and Estrada 2022).

The movement toward the modern era of medical simulation began in the 1960s. At the beginning of the decade, a toy manufacturer named Ausmund Laerdal worked alongside anesthesiologists to design a simulator to teach mouth-to-mouth ventilation. The mannequin became "Resusci-Anne" and revolutionized resuscitation training with a low-cost, readily available, effective training model (Bradley 2006; Cooper and Taqueti 2008; Jones et al. 2015). An internal spring was later attached to the mannequin's chest wall, permitting simulation of cardiac compressions. In 1968, Dr. Michael Gordon presented "Harvey," a cardiology patient simulator, to the American Heart Association (Jones et al. 2015).

Around the same time, another type of simulation was being developed. In 1963, Howard Barrows, a young academic neurologist, began to use actors to simulate neurological signs and symptoms in lessons with his students (Jones et al. 2015). Patient actors, more commonly termed *standardized patients (SPs)*, are now the most widely used simulation mode in medical education. Significant technological improvements throughout the 1980s and 1990s ushered in software and computerized systems that could be added to educational scenarios to mimic physiologic responses and provide real-time feedback. One of these systems (Gaba and colleagues' CASE simulator) would marry a Macintosh computer, a mannequin, and waveform generators to simulate the anesthesia process (Cooke et al. 2006). The year 2007 saw several medical schools develop and use "Second Life," a virtual reality, internet-based platform giving medical students a way to practice history-taking and clinical examination (Jones et al. 2015). These advancements in SBME are summarized and outlined in Table 17.1.

Most medical schools and residency programs have integrated formal simulation programs into their curricula. "Doctoring" courses routinely make use of SP interviews for both learning and assessment (Hawkins et al. 2012; Wang 2011). Standardized patient assessments are such an integral part of modern medical education assessment that before its cancellation in 2021, the United States Medical Licensing Examination (USMLE) Step 2 Clinical Skills (CS) Examination—the national standardized exam that assesses medical students' skills, physical exam aptitude, and professionalism—used SPs for each encounter. While Step 2 CS is no longer being administered, the onus is now on medical schools to determine how they will assess competency in the areas Step 2 CS did previously. It is hard to imagine how standardized patients will not continue to play an integral role in this process. Although SPs are one of the most used types of simulation in medical

Table 17.1 Historical examples of simulation-based medical education

Year	Examples	Developer	Technology
1911	Ms. Chase	Hartford Hospital	Low-technology
1958	Resusci-Anne	Asmund Laerdal	Low-technology
1963	Standardized patients	Howard Barrows	Simulated/standardized patient
1968	Harvey	Michael Gordon	Low-technology
1987	Comprehensive Anesthesia Simulation Environment (CASE 1.2)	David Gaba and colleagues	Complex task trainer
2007	Second Life	Multiple medical schools	Virtual reality
2009	SimMan 3G (human patient simulator)	Laerdal Corp.	High-fidelity patient simulator

education, many other simulation methods are used today, from low-technology anatomical models to high-fidelity patient simulators.

Educational Theory

> "He who studies medicine without books sails an uncharted sea, but he who studies medicine without patients does not go to sea at all."
>
> —William Osler

Traditionally, the preclinical phase of medical school is devoted to didactic teaching, and the clinical years of medical school and most residencies focus on experiential learning. Experiential learning is acknowledged as the cornerstone of medical education, in which direct experience is thought to be more educational than just didactics (Levine et al. 2013). However, real-time experiential learning is complex in busy wards and clinics, and interacting with patients as a new student can be daunting. SBME allows experiential learning to occur in a low-risk setting with many opportunities for observation and feedback.

Integrating simulation in the preclinical curriculum provides experiential learning sessions to complement classroom didactics. For residents and clinical-year students, simulation allows experiential learning to occur in a structured, standardized format. In these scenarios, there are three phases: preparation (prework, orientation, discussion of expectations), simulation activity, and debriefing (processing of the experience, feedback, and further education) (Chernikova et al. 2020). Unlike learning in clinical settings, this structured environment allows for a clear goal and expectations, a safe and predictable environment, and built-in time for detailed feedback and debriefing. Time constraints and the myriad complexities of patient care make directed learning more difficult. Additionally, active experimentation is easily accomplished in SBME because trainees can practice the same scenario repeatedly.

In recent years, emphasis has shifted to person-centered care. Thus students must know how to evaluate and treat various conditions and also how to approach a person as a whole and address complex problems that may influence their care. Simulated teaching allows for integrating this complexity without the unpredictable nature of clinical care experiences. It also shifts the teaching model from a didactic, paternalistic model to a collaborative, active learning experience.

Students are empowered to engage with the material and test their knowledge in a low-risk space (Chernikova et al. 2020).

Simulation Modalities

See Table 17.2 for the characteristics of the different modalities used in SBME.

Use of Simulation-Based Medical Education in Psychiatry

Simulation is widely used in all medical education, including psychiatry. As of 2011, about 45% of medical schools and 12% of teaching hospitals reported incorporating simulation in the psychiatry clerkship for medical students (Passiment et al. 2011). More than 20% of medical schools and 5% of teaching hospitals used simulation in psychiatry residency curricula. In an updated survey from 2020, 148 schools reported using simulation, and 151 schools used standardized patients, although more detailed breakdowns were unavailable (Association of American Medical Colleges 2025).

Psychiatry was a late adopter of SBME, but its implementation has rapidly expanded (Levine et al. 2013). SP encounters are by far the most used simulation type in psychiatric education (Abdool et al. 2017), although exploration of telehealth-based and virtual simulation methods is increasing. Here, we discuss these methods in greater detail.

Use of Standardized Patients

Standardized patients are widely used to teach trainees interview skills. Given that interviewing is the principal exam skill of psychiatrists, structured practice of patient interactions is a mainstay of education. SP interviews are beneficial for exposing students to a broad range of psychopathology and simulating high-risk scenarios such as suicidal patients (Brenner 2009). Frequently, SPs help students learn the content and structure of the mental status examination (Levine et al. 2013) and help residents practice psychotherapy (Coyle et al. 1998; Klamen and Yudkowsky 2002). Additionally, exposure to these exercises can help reduce the stigma of mental health conditions. Finally, learning how to interact with psychiatric patients in a controlled environment removes

Table 17.2 Characteristics of different simulation modalities

Simulation modality	Description	Applicable competencies	Limitations in psychiatric education	Resource requirements
Low-technology models	Anatomical models Inert mannequins	Anatomical knowledge Procedural skills	Limited applications in psychiatry Limited ability to respond to trainee input	Lower start-up and maintenance costs Instructor needed for any substantial feedback
Role-play	Enacting various scenarios and practicing how one would respond	Patient interview skills	Difficult to portray various conditions without appropriate training	Instructor and educational materials needed
Standardized patients	Actors or laypersons trained to portray patient scenarios	Patient interview skills, including those involving complex conversation Physical examination skills Professionalism Crisis management	Limited ability to teach complex interpersonal skills because of the explicit falseness of the scenario Difficulty simulating abnormal physical exam findings Variable reliability depending on experience, skill, SP training, and case number, length, and order Demonstrated relationship between experience with SPs and OSCE scores suggests practice effect or test-taking behavior	SP salaries High administrative costs for recruiting and training SPs Significant faculty time required for writing cases, facilitating teaching sessions, and evaluating performance on OSCEs

Table 17.2 Characteristics of different simulation modalities *(continued)*

Simulation modality	Description	Applicable competencies	Limitations in psychiatric education	Resource requirements
Screen-based computer simulation	Interactive computer programs that return different outputs based on trainee input that may involve AI	Patient interview skills Clinical decision-making Crisis management	Preprogrammed actions and responses; not adaptable Limited ability to teach and evaluate interpersonal skills	Expensive to develop or purchase Ongoing costs: equipment maintenance and software upgrades
Complex task trainers	Anatomical or surgical models integrated with computer programs to provide high-fidelity procedural training	Procedural skills	Limited applications in psychiatry	Expensive systems (>$15K) Ongoing costs: other equipment beyond that included with the model, equipment maintenance, and software upgrades
High-fidelity patient simulators	Mannequins integrated with computer systems, typically capable of simulating physical exam findings (e.g., pulse, breathing sounds) and displaying other relevant information (e.g., patient demographics, lab results)	Physical examination skills Clinical decision-making Crisis management Teamwork	Not capable of complex conversations	Costly systems (~$250K)

Table 17.2 Characteristics of different simulation modalities *(continued)*

Simulation modality	Description	Applicable competencies	Limitations in psychiatric education	Resource requirements
Virtual reality	Interactive system with sensory input (e.g., audiovisual, tactile) combined with user receptors (e.g., head or body trackers)	Patient interview skills Physical examination skills Clinical decision-making Crisis management Teamwork Procedural skills Interpersonal skills	Preprogrammed responses; not adaptable Limited nonverbal communication cues Faculty evaluator required	Limited existing programs and templates High start-up costs

Source. Brenner 2009; Chernikova et al. 2020; Cleland et al. 2009; Gaba 2004; Hall et al. 2004; Hawkins et al. 2012; Krahn et al. 2002; Levine et al. 2013; Patrício et al. 2013; Srinivasan et al. 2006; Stevens et al. 2006; Talente et al. 2007; Williams et al. 2011.

OSCE = observed structured clinical examination; SP = standardized patient.

the possible ethical and safety issues involved with direct patient care (Amsalem et al. 2020). Indeed, students who had one training course with an SP were shown to have improved psychiatric clinical skills and increased self-confidence (Amsalem et al. 2020).

SP interactions can be used to assess trainee competencies in psychiatry, from the mental status examination to suicide risk assessment (Hodges et al. 2014; Hung et al. 2012). OSCEs are a standard method for evaluating students' interview skills in the psychiatry clerkship (Brenner 2009). Objective checklist items and subjective measurements are used to evaluate the trainee's interpersonal skills, and they may be scored by faculty or SPs (Levine et al. 2013). Two studies have shown that OSCE scores correlate well with other trainee assessments, such as preceptor evaluations on inpatient wards (McLay et al. 2002; Whelan et al. 2009). For both faculty and SP scores, reliability is increased with a greater number and variety of OSCE stations (Swanson and van der Vleuten 2013); 6–10 observations per domain has been suggested for reliable assessment (Srinivasan et al. 2006).

Aside from evaluation, students find it helpful to work on their psychiatric skills with SPs. A small study surveyed students after they completed a simulation activity with SPs during their psychiatric rotation. Students felt like they learned practical skills in psychiatric interviews; they also felt like they could practice empathic communication. The simulation activity was perceived as "motivating" and did not cause additional stress (Siemerkus et al. 2023).

As SPs are increasingly used in psychiatric education, some authors have cautioned educators to be mindful of the limitations of SPs in teaching and assessing complex interpersonal skills. In psychiatry, SPs may find it especially difficult to portray pathology realistically. Furthermore, specific complex skills in psychiatry are inherently challenging to practice in a fabricated encounter, such as teasing out delusions from deliberate lies or recognizing truths that the patient has not yet explicitly acknowledged (Brenner 2009). Brenner suggests that SPs are most effective in teaching and assessing "discrete skills," such as covering all components of the mental status examination, rather than complex interpersonal skills (e.g., emotional responsiveness and empathy) (Brenner 2009).

Use of Mannequin-Based Simulation

Given the nature of psychiatric care, SPs are used more frequently during simulation exercises. However, mannequins can be useful for practicing medical emergencies in psychiatry, where it is important to recognize vital signs changes and other acute concerns. Some simulated scenarios have included lithium toxicity and alcohol withdrawal (Bhalla et al. 2017) and opioid overdose (where the patient responds to naloxone) (Baker et al. 2021). At the Medical University of South Carolina (MUSC), mannequins are used for several cases of delirium, specifically a case involving neuroleptic malignant syndrome. Using the mannequin and the monitors allows students to respond to changes in vital signs and lab findings; the interventions students choose are put into the simulation computer by a proctor, and the patient's status changes in response. Although the use of mannequins has been limited in psychiatric simulation, they can be a safe and cost-effective alternative to SPs, and they allow students to practice cases with high medical acuity in a safe and controlled environment (Baker et al. 2021).

Use of Screen-Based Computer Simulation

Computer simulations of the psychiatric interview were discussed in the literature as early as 1967 (Starkweather et al. 1967), but applications have remained limited. An early example from Beutler and Harwood (2004) piloted a psychotherapy simulation with a two-dimensional virtual patient displayed on a computer screen. As the trainee talked to the display, a trained observer categorized the trainee's questions or interventions and chose the appropriate preprogrammed response for the virtual patient based on branching logic. Another group developed a web-based simulation that involved selecting actions from multiple-choice lists to assess psychiatry residents' competency in obtaining informed consent for antipsychotic medications (Gorrindo et al. 2011). During pilot testing, residents reported that this simulation was easy to use and helped increase their confidence in acquiring informed consent (Gorrindo et al. 2011).

Evidence for computer-based case simulations for medical school has remained limited, however. Specifically, the validity of assessing decision-making skills in virtual patient case scenarios has been raised as a concern (Ward et al. 2019). Furthermore, computer simulations of psychiatric encounters are limited in their ability to portray complex social interactions realistically. Each response must be preprogrammed, and creating adaptable and detailed scripts to simulate a psychiatric interview is challenging. In the future, artificial intelligence (AI) software such as ChatGPT may also be able to respond and interact with students like a standardized patient (Okan 2023). For example, some medical universities in Germany have designed a program called "Medical TrAIning" that integrates virtual reality, faculty designed cases, and AI-related responses to trainees (Mergen et al. 2023). Other similar programs have been designed as well: studies examining improvement in clinical decision-making and interview skills have been promising (Bottrighi et al. 2025; Holderried et al. 2024; Kanazawa et al. 2023). It has also been suggested that AI could be used to create simulation programs themselves, although these programs should continue to be carefully vetted to avoid inclusion of erroneous information (Xu et al. 2024). AI software is advancing at a fast pace; with refined technology and appropriate programming, programs such as ChatGPT are likely to be a new cornerstone in virtual simulation.

Computers can be used for medical student education in other ways. Telehealth training is a particularly promising application for virtual patients. During the public health emergency due to COVID-19 in 2020, telehealth programs were rapidly initiated to ensure that patients received appropriate care, and many patients continue to be seen via telehealth. Therefore, students should learn how to interact with patients through videoconferencing. Guidelines for telehealth simulation have been published, including education about maintaining privacy and legal compliance (Martin et al. 2022). Telehealth has also been studied specifically for psychiatry, including important skills such as suicide risk assessment (Liew et al. 2022). The simulation involved a suicidal patient at home who could terminate the call at any time. Students did not meet three telemedicine competencies (establishing rapport, environmental assessment, and problem-based evaluation). It was determined that even though medical students are considered very tech-savvy, they should still receive formal education on conducting telehealth visits (Liew et al. 2022).

Use of High-Fidelity Patient Simulators and Virtual Reality

Virtual patients have been used in medical education to assess history-taking skills and practice delivering bad news. Virtual encounters are more effective if they include other supporting materials, such as presimulation tutorials, supportive prompts during the virtual encounter, and follow-up evaluations. Feedback could be generated by the system or provided by a proctor (Lee et al. 2020). In primary care, game-based patient simulations helped providers screen for mental health concerns, practice motivational interviewing, and learn how to integrate mental health care into their daily practice (Albright et al. 2013). Going forward, improving virtual patients' body language and overall quality will be key (Stewart and Mashmous 2023). Virtual reality systems also offer the unique opportunity to track trainee gaze direction and body positioning (Stevens et al. 2006), which could help provide feedback on nonverbal signaling during psychiatric interviews.

Simulation and the COVID-19 Pandemic

In 2020, medical education went through a significant upheaval. Patient care exposure was the primary way students traditionally learned in their clinical years. During the pandemic, the safety of students and patients was at risk. Clinical exposure was significantly limited for many types of learners in psychiatry. Telehealth and simulation tools became more important than ever to provide students with valuable clinical experience (Mitra and Fluyau 2023). Simulated patients and role-play helped students learn to navigate complex interactions and test their skills with psychiatric evaluation; these skills were of particular value in the public health emergency. Some focus points have included behavioral emergencies (agitated patients requiring de-escalation), relevant medical emergencies (neuroleptic malignant syndrome [NMS] and serotonin syndrome), and communication/interpersonal skills in psychiatric emergencies. Simulated patients, even video/simulated telepsychiatry, may be helpful (Mitra and Fluyau 2023). Additionally, simulated environments help students practice empathetic interactions with patients and work on teamwork and communication (Mitra and Fluyau 2023).

A combination of computer-accessed and in-person simulation has been examined as well (Tong et al. 2021). One study examined hybrid education in emergencies for psychiatric hospitalists and emergency providers. The goal was to educate them on psychiatric emergencies (such as NMS, medically ill patients with anorexia, and psychotic patients) and help avoid unnecessary complications. To accommodate COVID-19 concerns, the simulation was both held in person and broadcast to participants via Zoom. SPs were in the simulation center and connected to vitals-monitoring equipment when appropriate. Most participants, including those engaged virtually, found the course helpful. It was noted that this modality might be beneficial for educating remote or rural physicians (Tong et al. 2021).

Other Applications for Simulation

Beyond teaching and assessment, simulation has been used to foster understanding and empathy for patients among trainees (Levine et al. 2013). The most common application is using voice recordings, often based on patients' real hallucinations, to simulate auditory hallucinations for students (Levine et al. 2013). Previously, Yellowlees and Cook (2006) piloted an internet-based virtual reality system to simulate the audio and visual hallucinations of a person with schizophrenia. More recently, a more formal virtual reality simulation of psychotic patients' experiences has been used to promote empathy and reduce stigma among mental health providers (Riches et al. 2022).

Financing for Simulation Programs

There are several practical considerations when starting a simulation program. Expenses can be divided into direct costs (space, technology, supplies, salary for faculty and SPs) and indirect costs (administration, utilities, maintenance of space). Lost money, such as time attendings would otherwise see patients, should also be considered, particularly in hospital environments that prioritize relative value unit (RVU) generation. Funding can be obtained from institutional support, grants, and charged services provided to outside health care workers. Ongoing expenses can make sustaining a simulation center difficult, so expenses and revenue should be managed carefully to ensure ongoing operation (Senvisky et al. 2023).

There is limited information regarding specific simulation center costs; it is unclear whether the studies that have been published were transparent about all costs or whether the cost expectations were generalizable across programs. The benefit of academic institutions (particularly in economically advanced countries such as the United States) is that simulation centers may already exist at the institution, and different departments can access this pooled resource rather than putting forth significant expenses for a department-specific simulation center. However, given ongoing financial pressures in health care, it will be increasingly important for simulation centers to justify their benefit to continue receiving funding (Hippe et al. 2020). It is difficult to assess the full clinical benefits for patients (lives saved or more effective and efficient care) or downstream cost savings, particularly in psychiatry. There are no specific studies regarding the cost of psychiatric simulation.

In the AAMC survey on simulation programs, the annual operating budgets reported by medical schools were evenly split between the different budget categories (from $0–250,000 to >$1,000,000) (Passiment et al. 2011). Respondents varied widely in the types of administrative costs they included. An updated report is pending and will help determine simulation center costs. As of July 2025, results of a 2024 survey are still pending. However, data have been collected from 117 respondents covering more than 40 questions, including current and future planned use of simulation, accreditation, available simulation modalities, and information about types of learners, content, and assessed competencies (Association of American Medical Colleges 2025).

Eighty-four percent of medical schools and 90% of teaching hospitals reported complete or partial ownership of their simulation facilities. The most commonly reported funding sources were the medical school (87%), grants (40%), and courses and services to groups and individuals (33%) (Passiment et al. 2011). Most medical schools and hospitals (90% overall) reported sharing the simulation facilities with other health professionals and even nonclinical entities, such as industry (Passiment et al. 2011).

Current Evidence on Outcomes and Benefits

Research has shown that simulation in psychiatry education improves educational outcomes, including adherence to interview protocols and assessment scores (Hayes-Roth et al. 2010; Williams et al. 2017). Trainees reported that SP activities in psychiatry education are useful and satisfying (Brown et al. 2005; Hall et al. 2004). Simulation, including web-based experiences, can also help trainees and general population members understand and empathize with psychiatric symptoms (Ballon et al. 2007; Yellowlees and Cook 2006). Evidence is limited for more distant impacts. Outside of psychiatry, studies have shown that SBME is associated with positive outcomes at multiple translational levels, including in patient care practices, patient outcomes, and collateral effects such as cost savings (McGaghie et al. 2014).

A 2020 meta-analysis of 145 studies also examined how different simulation structures and technologies help with complex skill development. The analysis aimed to include simulation in all higher education, but medical education was most represented (126 of 145 studies). The analysis found that simulations fostered more complex skills than other teaching modalities, followed by some benefits in communication and situation management. The most effective types were SPs or a blend of SPs and virtual content. Mannequins and virtual reality were more useful than screen-based testing (Chernikova et al. 2020).

Quality-improvement studies have also examined how organized simulation activities help improve the safety and quality of care in hospital settings. For example, teams that ran simulations of codes had increased survival rates and a higher percentage of patients who achieved return of spontaneous circulation. In conditions where simulations were run in the hospital setting, teams could identify skill deficiencies and weak points in the system, improving overall care (Rider and Schertzer 2022). Although the quality improvement situations in this study were not identical to the training students get in medical school, it is clear that physical practice of skills in a controlled environment can better prepare all providers for performance in real-world conditions.

Case Study on Unstable Patient Simulation

Since 2009, all medical students at the Medical University of South Carolina (MUSC) have participated in an unstable patient simulation on a high-fidelity patient simulator during their third-year psychiatry clerkship (Funk et al. 2015). The simulation center at MUSC opened in June 2008 and was funded by donors to improve patient safety. In 2023, MUSC opened a new simulation center with updated mannequins and equipment and improved education spaces.

The primary focus of simulation for psychiatry at MUSC is medical emergencies in psychiatry, such as NMS or alcohol withdrawal/delirium tremens. Mannequins and vital signs monitors are used in these cases. Before each session, students are assigned background reading and quizzes. Groups of four to six students work together to talk with the patient, assess vitals and lab results, and make clinical decisions. A resident, attending, or a team of two people, provide feedback and act as the patient, family members, or staff. Specifically, the attending psychiatrist serves as the attending on-call, available by phone to the student team. Students are encouraged to interact as if the mannequin is the patient and reach out to collateral if this would be helpful. The psychiatry resident provides the voiceover for the mannequin and enters decisions into the computer that reflect the choices made by the students. This feeds into an algorithm that triggers changes in vital signs patient status (for example, the patient having a seizure in undertreated alcohol withdrawal). Once the session is complete, debriefing and education are provided. The session is not graded; it is treated as a learning experience.

Our case highlights an important point: suspension of disbelief (to a degree) is required in SBME, mainly regarding time (Herrera-Aliaga and Estrada 2022). Our time for the simulation (approximately 20 minutes) is insufficient to capture all the elements we hope to teach students (e.g., the frequency of giving additional lorazepam in alcohol withdrawal). This is an important part of the debriefing process, and we may provide time cues during the simulation so that students are aware of the amount of time that has elapsed since a previous event.

The simulation team has continued to modify the education experience based on teaching opportunities and feedback. During the case, a wider cast of characters has been added, including on-call nursing, the attending on-call, and family members who provide additional information. In addition to the case itself, instructions about capacity and commitment criteria have been added. Students are frequently exposed to these during their rotations, but the case provides formal education that will be practical for any field in which they specialize. The goal is to provide an educational experience in a relaxed environment where students can ask questions and make decisions.

Recommendations for Incorporating Simulation in Psychiatric Education

Content and Competencies

In psychiatry, simulation is beneficial for teaching and assessing discrete interview skills such as completing the mental status examination and managing unstable patients. As other authors have expounded (Brenner 2009), simulation is not well suited to teach interpersonal skills, although some exercises have been developed to foster empathy and reduce stigma.

Appropriate resources should be devoted to researching, writing, and piloting simulation cases. The development of prereading materials, patient and preceptor scripts, and teaching points is important to ensure a valuable and consistent learning experience. Focusing on specific skills and goals (such as mental status examination and safety planning) can keep the learning experience clear and ensure that students can practice needed skills. As noted earlier, simulated environments can also provide safe and structured exposure to emergent situations, such as acutely suicidal patients.

Educators should view simulation as an opportunity for interprofessional training. In health care settings, teams usually include members from different fields, specialties, and training levels, yet training remains siloed. Preclinical trainees are typically segregated by discipline, and although clinical trainees work on interdisciplinary teams, they rarely have integrated training or education sessions. Simulation offers an ideal opportunity to practice teamwork in high-risk scenarios. Simulation centers are exceptionally well suited for collaborative training because they are often jointly funded by different schools and departments.

Simulation Modalities

Standardized patients remain the preferred modality for scenarios with complex social interaction, since all other technologies remain limited in their ability to simulate realistic conversation. This is especially true if the SPs are emulating a complicated psychiatric scenario (such as acute suicide risk). Conversely, mannequin-based scenarios are useful for cases with physiologic findings (e.g., unstable vital signs, critical lab results), especially since the computer algorithms can adjust the patient's response to chosen interventions. Furthermore, remote simulation with SPs has also been used since the COVID-19 emergency to provide exposure to patient care while keeping both patients and students safe, and it could also be used to train providers in remote areas.

Computer-based simulations are best suited for discrete interview skills and clinical decision-making algorithms, especially since many of the nuances of patient care are lost in this decision-tree format. Virtual reality also holds the potential to provide immersive simulated experiences and will be especially useful for competencies in clinical decision-making and crisis management, although it is still under development. More importantly, virtual reality systems have also shown potential for fostering empathy in providers by simulating patient experiences. Advances in artificial intelligence are expected in the next decade and will likely become more widely used in simulation.

Therefore, faculty should monitor the variety of simulation modalities available for training.

Simulation Activity Structure

Before the simulation activity, students should be provided with appropriate prework materials to prepare them for the simulation content. Before the simulation begins, students should be oriented to the simulation center functions (as applicable), and clear expectations should be laid out. After the simulation activity has been completed, debriefing should always take place. Students should be given feedback, and relevant learning points should be reinforced. Debriefing facilitates the reflective observation stage of Kolb's experiential learning cycle (Levine et al. 2013) and is recognized as crucial for the effectiveness of simulation-based learning (Issenberg et al. 2005).

For most simulations, immersion and believability will be improved by having minimal instructor interjections during the activity. To ensure a complete learning experience, however, some feedback can be provided in real time to help the simulation run smoothly. In our experience, incorporating an attending on-call role can minimize student frustration and prevent them from making egregious mistakes that would end the simulation scenario abruptly.

If time and equipment resources are limited, having groups of trainees participate in the simulation is feasible and has some benefits over individual participation. Working in a group can reduce pressure on the individual student, minimize trainee embarrassment, allow teamwork practice, and encourage interprofessional collaboration. However, students may also feel anxious and embarrassed in front of their peers, and it can be more challenging to engage each student when simulations are done in a group. One way to work around this is to provide each student with a specific role and expectations.

Simulation Program Funding

In many institutions in the United States, simulation centers are already accessible, although different departments will require different resources. There are still many expenses to consider for the institution and individual departments that help pay for the center. Using SPs requires the infrastructure and funds for training, recruiting, and salaries. Other simulation types may have higher up-front development costs and ongoing equipment maintenance and software upgrade expenses. For all simulation types, administrative costs for running the program cannot be overlooked. Evaluating the ongoing costs of simulation centers is important to ensure their viability. Grants may help start a program, but sustainability must be well thought through.

Discussion and Conclusions

Providing a graduating escalation of responsibility as students progress is difficult in traditional medical training. For airplane pilots, training often incorporates a ride-along instructor who can take control of the flight anytime. Conversely, medical training does not allow for such close supervision or the ability for a supervisor to assume control of the situation seamlessly. This is especially true in psychiatry, where most of the work happens during the interview between the patient and trainee.

SBME allows learners to take on more significant degrees of responsibility in low-risk settings, provides time for reflection and feedback, and allows repetitive practice. When simulation activities are immersive and realistic, they facilitate substantial experiential learning. Simulation also allows for structured, standardized assessments. Because of these advantages, simulation has been hailed as a method for improving trainee competence and patient safety. Research shows positive impacts at multiple levels of translational outcomes for general SBME, although data are more limited in psychiatry education.

Going forward, we expect to see greater incorporation of computer-based simulation, high-fidelity patient simulators, AI, and virtual reality simulations in SBME, especially as these technologies improve and become more accessible. The COVID-19 emergency also forced programs to be more creative in exposing students to patient care, and simulation grew to be especially useful. Artificial intelligence may one day replace the branching logic used in most simulation methods so that the range of possible reactions and scenarios is not limited by what was preprogrammed. This could allow systems to respond fluidly to trainee input and realistically simulate conversation, which is currently a significant deficiency in all simulations that do not involve SPs. With the advent of ChatGPT, there has been some speculation regarding its use in simulating patient experiences, although data do not currently exist.

Simulation provides an ideal setting for practicing team dynamics, but currently, there is little published experience in incorporating interprofessional teams into psychiatric simulations. This would be especially useful in training teams to respond to mental health crises, such as the severely agitated patient. This has the potential to improve safety for both patients and health care providers. We hope to see more research and reports on this topic.

In psychiatry, there has been limited research on how SBME programs impact more distant implementation outcomes, especially care practices and patient outcomes. Improving patient safety is a key goal of simulation programs, and demonstrating evidence would help secure and justify funding for simulation programs.

Simulation is an important component of medical education. Although psychiatry has lagged behind other fields in its implementation, it has become a cornerstone of training for medical students and residents. It provides a safe, controlled environment for students to practice specific skills and receive real-time feedback. In psychiatry specifically, it is helpful for honing interview skills and responding to emergencies. Depending on the institution, simulation centers can be expensive and difficult to access. Continued improvement of remote, computer- and virtual-based simulations will help provide educational resources to providers who may not have local access. Finally, simulation has excellent potential to improve teamwork in psychiatric care. More detailed studies are needed to understand the impact simulated training has on patient care.

Key Points

- Simulation-based medical education (SBME) can offer students a supportive environment to learn, engage more directly in realistic problem-solving, and learn from experience in low-risk settings.
- Different simulation modalities are available, including computer-based simulations and standardized patients; some of the possible applications of SBME in psychiatry include practicing interview skills, exercising clinical decision-making and crisis management, and helping foster empathy.
- In psychiatry, there has been limited research on the impact of SBME programs, especially regarding care practices and patient outcomes.

References

Abdool P, Nirula L, Bonato S, et al: Simulation in undergraduate psychiatry: exploring the depth of learner engagement. Acad Psychiatry 41(2):251–261, 2017 27882523

Albright G, Adam C, Goldman R, Serri D: A game-based simulation utilizing virtual humans to train physicians to screen and manage the care of patients with mental health disorders. Games Health J 2(5):269–273, 2013 26196927

Amsalem D, Gothelf D, Soul O, et al: Single-day simulation-based training improves communication and psychiatric skills of medical students. Front Psychiatry 11:221, 2020 32265762

Armenia S, Thangamathesvaran L, Caine AD, et al: The role of high-fidelity team-based simulation in acute care settings: a systematic review. Surg J (NY) 4(3):e136–e151, 2018 30109273

Association of American Medical Colleges: Instructional Methods Used by Medical Schools. AAMC, 2011. Available at: https://www.aamc.org/data-reports/curriculum-reports/data/instructional-methods-used-medical-schools. Accessed July 30, 2023.

Association of American Medical Colleges: Medical Simulation in Medical Education. AAMC, 2025. Available at: https://www.aamc.org/about-us/mission-areas/medical-education/medical-simulation. Accessed July 11, 2025.

Baker SE, Escamilla K, Jacobs M, et al: Manikin-based simulation: an update to the clerkship experience. Acad Psychiatry 45(4):530–531, 2021 34008133

Ballon BC, Silver I, Fidler D: Headspace theater: an innovative method for experiential learning of psychiatric symptomatology using modified role-playing and improvisational theater techniques. Acad Psychiatry 31(5):380–387, 2007 17875623

Beutler LE, Harwood TM: Virtual reality in psychotherapy training. J Clin Psychol 60(3):317–330, 2004 14981794

Bhalla IP, Wilkins KM, Moadel T, et al: Alcohol withdrawal and lithium toxicity: a novel psychiatric mannequin-based simulation case for medical students. MedEdPORTAL 13:10649, 2017 30800850

Bottrighi A, Grosso F, Ghiglione M, et al: A symbolic AI approach to medical training. J Med Syst 49(1):1–15, 2025

Bradley P: The history of simulation in medical education and possible future directions. Med Educ 40(3):254–262, 2006 16483328

Brenner AM: Uses and limitations of simulated patients in psychiatric education. Acad Psychiatry 33(2):112–119, 2009 19398623

Brown R, Doonan S, Shellenberger S: Using children as simulated patients in communication training for residents and medical students: a pilot program. Acad Med 80(12):1114–1120, 2005 16306284

Buck GH: Development of simulators in medical education. Gesnerus 48(Pt 1):7–28, 1991 1855669

Campbell KK, Wong KE, Kerchberger AM, et al: Simulation-based education in US undergraduate medical education: a descriptive study. Simul Healthc 18(6):359-366, 2023 36584239

Chernikova O, Heitzmann N, Fisher F: Simulation-based learning in higher education: a meta-analysis. Rev Educ Res 90(4):499–541, 2020

Cleland JA, Abe K, Rethans J-J: The use of simulated patients in medical education: AMEE Guide No 42. Med Teach 31(6):477–486, 2009 19811162

Cook DA, Brydges R, Zendejas B, et al: Mastery learning for health professionals using technology-enhanced simulation: a systematic review and meta-analysis. Acad Med 88(8):1178–1186, 2013 23807104

Cooke M, Irby DM, Sullivan W, Ludmerer KM: American medical education 100 years after the Flexner report. N Engl J Med 355(13):1339–1344, 2006 17005951

Cooper JB, Taqueti VR: A brief history of the development of mannequin simulators for clinical education and training. Postgrad Med J 84(997):563–570, 2008 19103813

Coyle B, Miller M, McGowen KR: Using standardized patients to teach and learn psychotherapy. Acad Med 73(5):591–592, 1998 9643906

Funk M, Pelic C, Pelic C, et al: Simulation Centers in Consultation-Liaison Psychiatry Education: A Practical Workshop. Presented at Academy of Psychosomatic Medicine, 2015 Annual Meeting, New Orleans

Gaba DM: The future vision of simulation in health care. Qual Saf Health Care 13(Suppl 1):i2–i10, 2004 15465951

Gorrindo T, Baer L, Sanders KM, et al: Web-based simulation in psychiatry residency training: a pilot study. Acad Psychiatry 35(4):232–237, 2011 21804041

Hall MJ, Adamo G, McCurry L, et al: Use of standardized patients to enhance a psychiatry clerkship. Acad Med 79(1):28–31, 2004 14690994

Hawkins SC, Osborne A, Schofield SJ, et al: Improving the accuracy of self-assessment of practical clinical skills using video feedback—the importance of including benchmarks. Med Teach 34(4):279–284, 2012 22455696

Hayes-Roth B, Saker R, Amano K: Automating individualized coaching and authentic role-play practice for brief intervention training. Methods Inf Med 49(4):406–411, 2010 20405093

Herrera-Aliaga E, Estrada LD: Trends and innovations of simulation for twenty first century medical education. Front Public Health 10:619769, 2022 35309206

Hippe DS, Umoren RA, McGee A, et al: A targeted systematic review of cost analyses for implementation of simulation-based education in healthcare. SAGE Open Med 8:2050312120913451, 2020 32231781

Hodges B, Hollenberg E, McNaughton N, et al. The psychiatry OSCE: a 20-year retrospective. Acad Psychiatry 38(1):26–34, 2014 24449223

Holderried F, Stegemann-Phillips C, Herrmann-Werner A, et al: A language-model powered simulated patient with automated feedback for history taking: prospective study. JMIR Med Educ 10(e59213):1–14, 2024

Hung EK, Binder RL, Fordwood SR, et al: A method for evaluating competency in assessment and management of suicide risk. Acad Psychiatry 36(1):23–28, 2012 22362432

Institute of Medicine Committee on Quality of Health Care: To Err Is Human: Building a Safer Health System. Edited by Kohn LT, Corrigan JM, Donaldson MS. Washington, DC, National Academies Press, 2000

Issenberg SB, McGaghie WC, Petrusa ER, et al: Features and uses of high-fidelity medical simulations that lead to effective learning: a BEME systematic review. Med Teach 27(1):10–28, 2005 16147767

Jónasson JT: Educational change, inertia and potential futures. Eur J Futures Res 4(1):7, 2016

Jones F, Passos-Neto CE, Braghiroli OFM: Simulation in medical education: brief history and methodology. Principles Pract Clin Res 1(2), 2015

Kanazawa A, Fujibayashi K, Watanabe Y, et al: Evaluation of a medical interview-assistance system using artificial intelligence for resident physicians interviewing simulated patients: a crossover, randomized control trial. Int J Environ Res Public Health 20(6176):1–12, 2023

Klamen DL, Yudkowsky R: Using standardized patients for formative feedback in an introduction to psychotherapy course. Acad Psychiatry 26(3):168–172, 2002 12824134

Krahn LE, Bostwick JM, Sutor B, Olsen MW: The challenge of empathy: a pilot study of the use of standardized patients to teach introductory psychopathology to medical students. Acad Psychiatry 26(1):26–30, 2002 11867425

Lee Y, Kim SK, Eom M: Usability of mental illness simulation involving scenarios with patients with schizophrenia via immersive virtual reality. PLoS 15(9):e0238437, 2020

Lentz GM, Mandel LS, Goff BA: A six-year study of surgical teaching and skills evaluation for obstetric/gynecologic residents in porcine and inanimate surgical models. Am J Obstet Gynecol 193(6):2056–2061, 2005 16325615

Levine AI, DeMaria S Jr, Schwartz AD, Sim AJ (eds): The Comprehensive Textbook of Healthcare Simulation. New York, Springer, 2013

Liew A, Monkman H, Palmer R, et al: A Telepsychiatry Simulation for Suicide Assessment: Teaching Telemedicine Safety Competencies, in AMIA Annual Symposium Proceedings Archives, 2022, pp 700–708

Martin R, Mandrusiak A, Russell T, Forbes R: A toolbox for teaching telehealth using simulation. Clin Teach 19(4):270–275, 2022 35726556

McGaghie WC, Issenberg SB, Barsuk JH, Wayne DB: A critical review of simulation-based mastery learning with translational outcomes. Med Educ 48(4):375–385, 2014 24606621

McGaghie WC: Mastery learning: it is time for medical education to join the 21st century. Acad Med 90(11):1438–1441, 2015 26375269

McLay RN, Rodenhauser P, Anderson DS, et al: Simulating a full-length psychiatric interview with a complex patient: an OSCE for medical students. Acad Psychiatry 26(3):162–167, 2002 12824133

Mergen M, Junga A, Risse B, et al: Immersive training of clinical decision making with AI driven virtual patients—a new VR platform called Medical TrAIning. GMS J Med Educ 40(2):1–12, 2023

Mitra P, Fluyau D: The current role of simulation in psychiatry. Treasure Island, FL, StatPearls Publishing, 2023

Okan Ç: AI and psychiatry: the ChatGPT perspective. Alpha Psychiatry 24(2):41–42, 2023 37144055

Owen H: Early use of simulation in medical education. Simul Healthc 7(2):102–116, 2012 22374231

Passiment M, Sacks H, Huang G: Medical simulation in medical education: results of an AAMC survey. Association of American Medical Colleges, 2011. Available at: https://www.aamc.org/media/22586/download. Accessed July 12, 2025.

Patrício MF, Julião M, Fareleira F, Carneiro AV: Is the OSCE a feasible tool to assess competencies in undergraduate medical education? Med Teach 35(6):503–514, 2013 23521582

Piot MA, Attoe C, Billon G, et al: Simulation training in psychiatry for medical education: a review. Front Psychiatry 12:658967, 2021 34093275

Riches S, Iannelli H, Reynolds L, et al: Virtual reality-based training for mental health staff: a novel approach to increase empathy, compassion, and subjective understanding of service user experience. Adv Simul (Lond) 7(1):19, 2022 35854343

Rider A, Schertzer K: Quality improvement in medical simulation. Treasure Island, FL, StatPearls Publishing, 2022

Rosen KR: The history of medical simulation. J Crit Care 23(2):157–166, 2008 18538206

Schnorrenberger CC: Anatomical roots of Chinese medicine and acupuncture. Swiss J Integr Med 20(3):163, 2008

Senvisky JM, McKenna RT, Okuda Y: Financing and funding a simulation center. Treasure Island, FL, StatPearls Publishing, 2023

Siemerkus J, Petrescu AS, Köchli L, et al: Using standardized patients for undergraduate clinical skills training in an introductory course to psychiatry. BMC Med Educ 23(1):159, 2023 36922802

Sperling JD, Clark S, Kang Y: Teaching medical students a clinical approach to altered mental status: simulation enhances traditional curriculum. Med Educ Online 18(1):1–8, 2013 23561054

Srinivasan M, Hwang JC, West D, Yellowlees PM: Assessment of clinical skills using simulator technologies. Acad Psychiatry 30(6):505–515, 2006 17139022

Starkweather JA, Kamp M, Monto A: Psychiatric interview simulation by computer. Methods Inf Med 6(1):15–23, 1967 6043319

Stevens A, Hernandez J, Johnsen K, et al: The use of virtual patients to teach medical students history taking and communication skills. Am J Surg 191(6):806–811, 2006 16720154

Stewart CJ, Mashmous AB: Training for psychiatric assessments using virtual simulation. J Ment Health Train Educ Pract 18(3):261–273, 2023

Swanson DB, van der Vleuten CPM: Assessment of clinical skills with standardized patients: state of the art revisited. Teach Learn Med 25(S1):S17–S25, 2013

Talente G, Haist SA, Wilson JF: The relationship between experience with standardized patient examinations and subsequent standardized patient examination performance: a potential problem with standardized patient exam validity. Eval Health Prof 30(1):64–74, 2007 17293609

Tong K, McMahon E, Reid-McDermott B, et al: SafePsych: improving patient safety by delivering high-impact simulation training on rare and complex scenarios in psychiatry. BMJ Open Qual 10(3):e001533, 2021 34497099

Wang EE: Simulation and adult learning. Dis Mon 57(11):664–678, 2011 22082552

Ward RC, Muckle TJ, Kremer MJ, Krogh MA: Computer-based case simulations for assessment in health care: a literature review of validity evidence. Eval Health Prof 42(1):82–102, 2019 28727944

Whelan P, Church L, Kadry K: Using standardized patients' marks in scoring postgraduate psychiatry OSCEs. Acad Psychiatry 33(4):319–322, 2009 19690114

Wijnen-Meijer M, ten Cate O, van der Schaaf M, Harendza S: Graduates from vertically integrated curricula. Clin Teach 10(3):155–159, 2013 23656676

Williams B, Reddy P, Marshall S, et al: Simulation and mental health outcomes: a scoping review. Adv Simul (Lond) 2(1):2, 2017 29450003

Williams K, Wryobeck J, Edinger W, et al: Assessment of competencies by use of virtual patient technology. Acad Psychiatry 35(5):328–330, 2011 22007093

Xu X, Chen Y, Miao J: Opportunities, challenges, and future directions of large language models, including ChatGPT in medical education: a systematic scoping review. J Educ Eval Health Prof 21(6), 2024

Yellowlees PM, Cook JN: Education about hallucinations using an internet virtual reality system: a qualitative survey. Acad Psychiatry 30(6):534–539, 2006 17139026

Ziv A, Small SD, Wolpe PR: Patient safety and simulation-based medical education. Med Teach 22(5):489–495, 2000 21271963

Ziv A, Wolpe PR, Small SD, Glick S: Simulation-based medical education: an ethical imperative. Acad Med 78(8):783–788, 2003 12915366

Part IV

Special Themes in Undergraduate Psychiatric Education

18

Ethicolegal Considerations for Undergraduate Medical Educators

Jamie S. Padmore, D.M.
Steven A. Epstein, M.D.

Ethicolegal issues involving the oversight and management of medical students generally fall into two main categories: student performance and student health. In this chapter, we focus on the oversight of undergraduate medical education and the management of medical students enrolled in medical schools in the United States (we do not address the management of residents and fellows).

In this chapter, applicable federal laws, statutes, and regulations are defined and applied to faculty decision-making specific to student performance (academic performance and behavior, professional conduct). Likewise, decision-making specific to student medical and mental health issues is explored according to specific federal laws. As with any analysis, we define federal laws applicable to all schools and all students in the United States; care should be taken to recognize nuances subject to state or local regulation.

Laws, Statutes, and Regulations

Defining Due Process

> Mason, a medical student rotating on a 4-week psychiatry inpatient clerkship, was noted to have significant deficiencies in interviewing and conducting a mental status examination. At the rotation midpoint, Mason was given substantial (verbal) feedback on their deficiencies and suggestions on how to improve them. By the end of the rotation, they had improved only marginally. In addition, they scored in the third percentile on the national shelf exam in psychiatry. Mason was given a final grade of "failure" and was told they needed to repeat the rotation. Mason requested to appeal the failing grade.

Two Supreme Court decisions define the core tenets of due process as it is applied to academia. *Board of Curators of the University of Missouri v. Horowitz* (1978) established the criteria for academic due process. In this case, Ms. Horowitz was enrolled in the University of Missouri School of Medicine. Although she excelled during her first 2 years of basic science education, she received negative feedback (both verbal and written in rotational evaluations) when her clinical rotations began in her third year. She was criticized for her "poor bedside manner, bad hygiene, and slovenly appearance." Examples included acts considered "outrageous" by some at that time, including her refusal to wear a bra, not shaving under her arms, and not wearing deodorant. Despite this feedback, Horowitz did not change her behavior. The faculty at a "regularly scheduled meeting of the faculty to discuss student performance" agreed that Horowitz did not physically represent the role of a physician as was expected by the faculty at the time. Because she did not correct her behavior, the school dismissed her. Horowitz appealed to the dean, who in turn assigned her to rotate with seven independent physicians. Three of these physicians evaluated her as "acceptable," three evaluated her as "unacceptable," and the final physician said they could "go either way." Based on what the dean referred to as "consensus," he upheld the decision to dismiss Horowitz. She sued, citing discrimination (a charge that was eventually dropped) and lack of due process.

The Supreme Court heard the case on the sole allegation of lack of due process. The court ultimately sided with the university, noting that the school provided Horowitz with ample due process, defined as follows:

1. Horowitz was provided *notice* of her deficiencies through private verbal feedback and routine rotational evaluations.
2. Horowitz was provided an *opportunity to cure* her deficiencies.
3. The *decision was made carefully and deliberately.* The regularly called meeting of the faculty, called for the purpose of evaluating academic performance was noted as being a reasonable decision-making process consisting of faculty members charged with evaluating student performance.

Notice of her deficiencies were provided both verbally and in writing as part of the normal rotational evaluation process. The opportunity to cure was noted as reasonable given the circumstances for which she was criticized. Finally, the regular meeting of the faculty with the purpose of discussing student performance was noted to be a reasonable decision-making process. In their decision, the court noted that Horowitz actually received "much more process than was due," citing the meeting and review by the dean and the rotations with the seven independent physicians. In fact, either verbal feedback or the rotational evaluations would have sufficed in terms of "notice."

Horowitz ultimately defined the three core tenets of academic due process. Labor laws governing employers had already established due process as "notice, opportunity to be heard, and a reasonable decision-making process." This nuance, noting an opportunity to be heard (vs. an opportunity to cure) is the framework used for nonacademic due process (e.g., behavioral or conduct issues).

Board of Regents of the University of Michigan v. Ewing (1985) relied on *Horowitz* and added important legal context for academic decision-making. Mr. Ewing was enrolled in the 6-year BS/MD program at the University of Michigan in the early 1980s. After 4 years, he wrote the National Board Medical Examination (NBME) Part 1 exam and failed. Following this failure, he was dismissed from medical school. Ewing sued, citing at least 11 other students who previously failed the same examination but were allowed to remain enrolled and retake the test; some were allowed to retake the exam three or four times until they passed. In fact, Ewing was the only student in the history of the school who was dismissed after one such failure.

The school's faculty included a committee charged with reviewing academic performance of the students. This committee reviewed Ewing's entire academic record and concluded that his overall academic performance (which included several incompletes, required repeats of courses, and the lowest score ever recorded on the NBME at the school) did not indicate the ability or the aptitude required of a physician, and that he had no chance of ever succeeding.

The court sided with the school, noting the following:

1. The narrow avenue for judicial review of the substance of academic decisions precludes any conclusion that "such decision was a substantial departure from accepted academic norms as to demonstrate the faculty did not exercise professional judgment."
2. The decision-making process was "conscientious and made with careful deliberation," citing the regularly called meeting of the faculty, the Promotion and Review Board.
3. The faculty rightly reviewed Mr. Ewing's entire academic record, not just a single test rotation or incident, to provide context to their decision.

Together, these two Supreme Court decisions provide educators with a simple framework for making decisions specific to student performance (Table 18.1). In addition to the three core tenets of due process, *Ewing* allows education decision-makers to rely on a student's entire academic record to provide context in determining whether additional time or interventions may be an effective remedy for academic failure. The entire academic record includes any information available to the faculty, including performance in undergraduate studies and the entire performance record in medical school.

During the appeal process, Mason contended that at least two other students scored lower than the 5th percentile but were not required to retake the course. The appeal panel, however, noted that Mason was given *notice* of their deficiencies and *opportunity to cure*. The panel also

Table 18.1 **Due process standards: academic versus nonacademic matters**

Academic due process	Nonacademic due process (conduct)
1. Notice of (academic) deficiencies	1. Notice of charges or allegations
2. Opportunity to cure	2. Opportunity to be heard
3. Reasonable decision-making process	3. Reasonable decision-making process

> looked at Mason's entire academic record, which included related deficiencies in other specialties and at least two grades of "low pass." The panel noted that the negative feedback on interviewing skills was based on a consensus of several individuals, including two residents and a senior attending. Finally, the clerkship had notified all students at the beginning of the rotation that a score on the national exam above the 5th percentile was expected to pass the course. Thus, when considering all of the factors, the failing grade was upheld by the appeal panel.

Despite the expectation of scoring above the 5th percentile, each student's entire academic performance can (and should) be considered in the context of academic performance and decision-making, thus negating the employment concept of "similarly situated" (*Ewing*). Legally, allowing two other students to retake the exam and pass the course is not relevant to Mason's situation.

Health Insurance Portability and Accountability Act

> Abigail is a first-year medical student with a history of depression who is noticing signs of significantly increased stress and anxiety by the third month of classes. They recognize that test-taking is a trigger to stress and anxiety. They begin to regularly see a therapist in the university's student health center. They do not want to disclose their diagnosis of depression or anxiety to their medical school leaders or faculty, nor do they request any accommodations.

Overseen by the United States Department of Health and Human Services, the Health Insurance Portability and Accountability Act of 1996 (HIPAA) (Pub. L. No. 104-191) is a well-known federal law that sets a national standard to protect medical records and personal health information. Enacted in 1996, HIPAA excludes student medical records for health care provided by the university to currently enrolled students, deferring to the Family Educational Rights and Privacy Act (FERPA). HIPAA does apply to individuals who receive their care at the university but did not enroll as a student, or are no longer a student, in which case the university is then identified as a health care provider (Daggett 2019).

However, HIPAA specifically excludes student records with a wholesale exemption offering no differentiation as to whether a school is acting in a health care capacity (e.g., a medical school) or a purely educational capacity (Daggett 2019). This can be particularly confusing for both students and leaders when a medical school is concurrently operating in a health care capacity (e.g., running a hospital or health care facilities), allowing the school to provide clinical care services to enrolled students.

Family Educational Rights and Privacy Act

The Family Educational Rights and Privacy Act (FERPA) (Pub. L. No. 103-382, 20 U.S.C. § 1232g; 34 CFR Part 99) is a federal law protecting the privacy of student education records, inclusive of student health records. FERPA applies to schools (public, private, preschool, K–12, and postsecondary) receiving federal education funding and affords parents the right to access their children's education records, the right to seek to have records amended, and the right to have some control over the disclosure of personally identifiable information from records (https://studentprivacy.ed.gov/faq/what-ferpa) (U.S. Department of Education 2024).

There are several exceptions to the general consent requirements under FERPA. For example, institutions can disclose private information from a student's education records, including health and medical information, to faculty and other officials within the school, without prior written consent, if these school officials have been determined to have "legitimate educational interests" in the education records (https://studentprivacy.ed.gov/resources/joint-guidance-application-ferpa-and-hipaa-student-health-records). Institutions can also disclose private information from a student's education records, without prior written consent, to appropriate parties in connection with an emergency, if the parties' knowledge of the information is necessary to protect the health or safety of the student or other individuals.

Under FERPA, "treatment records," as they are commonly called, are excluded from the definition of "education records." Treatment records are defined as "records on a student who is eighteen years of age or older, or is attending an institution of postsecondary education, which are made or maintained by a physician, psychiatrist, psychologist, or other recognized professional or paraprofessional acting in his professional or paraprofessional capacity, or assisting in that capacity, and which are made, maintained, or used only in connection with the provision of treatment to the student, and are not available to anyone other than persons providing such treatment, except that such records can be personally reviewed by a physician or other appropriate professional of the student's choice" (20 U.S. Code § 1232g).

Institutions subject to both HIPAA and FERPA that operate clinics or other health care facilities open to staff, the public, or both (including family members of students) are required to comply with FERPA with respect to the health records ("education records" or "treatment records") of their student patients, and with HIPAA with respect to the health records of nonstudent patients. One consequence of this statute is that treatment records can be shared with other providers (off-campus) treating the student without the student's express consent. For example, a student with a chronic health condition, such as depression, and treated by a campus therapist may have their records shared with an off-campus third party without their express consent (Daggett 2019) unless university policies specify differently.

Application of Laws to Student Performance in Medical School

Academic Performance

When students fail to meet a school's academic standards, difficult decisions must be made regarding the continued enrollment of the student. Supreme Court rulings such as *Horowitz* and *Ewing* provide clarity of basic academic due-process requirements. However, the Liaison Commission for Medical Education (LCME) requires schools to have written policies. Often, in an effort to be thorough, schools develop lengthy policies that actually end up requiring standards higher than what the law mandates. Schools must follow their written policies. Lengthy policies can often lead to confusion or unintentional application, creating risk for the school. The majority of lawsuits filed in medical education include claims of lack of due process or discrimination (Minicucci and Lewis 2003).

The amount of time required for a student to improve should be reasonable based on the issue identified. As noted in *Horowitz*, "notice" does not need to be a formal construct, nor does it need to be objective; it may be subjective verbal feedback, routine evaluations, or a more structured (objective) assessment of performance. However, many schools have policies reminiscent of progressive discipline imposed by employers (constructs such as remediation or probation). These constructs are not required by any laws but are routinely implemented in medical school education and often extend into residency training, creating standards by institutional policy that are more onerous than what the law actually requires.

Likewise, medical schools have structures in place to assess student performance, often referred to as a "Committee for Progress and Promotions." Regardless of the name of the committee, a "regularly called meeting of the faculty for the purpose of assessing student performance" is one way of meeting the requirement of a "reasonable decision-making process" (Board of Curators of the University of Missouri v. Horowitz 1978; Board of Regents of the University of Michigan v. Ewing 1985). It should also be noted that performance decisions do not need to be made by majority, nor should a vote be taken. In *Horowitz*, the court noted support of the dean's decision to uphold the decision to dismiss based on consensus of the faculty, which was not unanimous. Voting provides a false sense of empowerment of a committee; instead, committee feedback should be provided to a decision-maker for determining appropriate action.

Student Conduct

> During a psychiatric rotation, Sam identified strongly with a vulnerable patient with borderline personality disorder who had been admitted after a suicide attempt. During the rotation, Sam was observed spending extra time with the patient after rounds. Later in the admission process, the patient reported to the attending psychiatrist that they wanted to leave against medical advice because of poor care that was pointed out to them by the student. When interviewed further, the patient also disclosed that the student had been texting with them frequently, and that they had agreed to meet for drinks after the patient was discharged.

This distinction between academic performance and conduct becomes particularly important in issues related to learners' behaviors. Whereas many performance deficiencies are purely academic (such as lack of knowledge or inability to apply it, inadequate judgment, or poor technical performance), others involve lapses in professional behavior or misconduct. Frohna and Padmore (2021) delineated the gray zone between the (academic) competency of professionalism and behavioral misconduct (Figure 18.1).

Schools should differentiate between professionalism as an *academic competency* versus professionalism issues that are *misconduct* (e.g., dishonesty). It is reasonable to expect that a college student knows lying is wrong (there is unlikely to be an educational intervention to teach someone not to be dishonest). Likewise, there is no assessment to ensure an intervention has succeeded and the student is no longer lying. Perhaps they do become truthful, or perhaps it is only that they are not caught. In cases of misconduct, programs must still ensure due process, but they do not have to extend an *opportunity to cure* that may enable recurrent misconduct and risk to the institution. The minimum requirement for due process in academic misconduct situations includes notice of the allegation, an opportunity to be heard on the allegation, and a reasonable process for deciding whether the learner engaged in misconduct.

Behaviors other than dishonesty, such as boundary violations with patients, can be more complex to evaluate and manage. In the earlier vignette, Sam was accused of significant boundary violation issues by a patient that were consistent with observations by others (e.g., spending extra time with the patient after rounds). It is always important to make sure the student has an opportunity to be heard before reaching any conclusions, regardless of how obvious things may seem based on an initial report.

When a student engages in improper behavior, it must be determined whether the action is misconduct or a breach of professionalism. Misconduct includes behaviors that a reasonable person would know are wrong (e.g., lying, cheating, stealing). When it is determined that the behavior was a mistake, however, or that it was something the individual shows the capacity to learn from (and not engage in again), it can be handled as an academic matter. To make this determination, the student should be told of the allegation made against them (*notice*) and allowed to speak on their own behalf (*opportunity to respond*). Based on the student's response to the allegation, especially if the student disagrees or contests the allegation, a subsequent inquiry may be necessary to determine what happened. This inquiry should be led by someone who is trained to facilitate such matters, such as human resources or the student affairs office. The inquiry can serve as the reasonable decision-making process as defined by the courts. Results of an inquiry should be provided to an appropriate decision-maker to determine next steps. If the student does not contest the allegation, then an inquiry may not need to take place.

Conducting an inquiry does not require irrefutable evidence. In fact, many times, the inquiry process may involve ambiguous or nuanced information from many sources. A misconduct inquiry is not

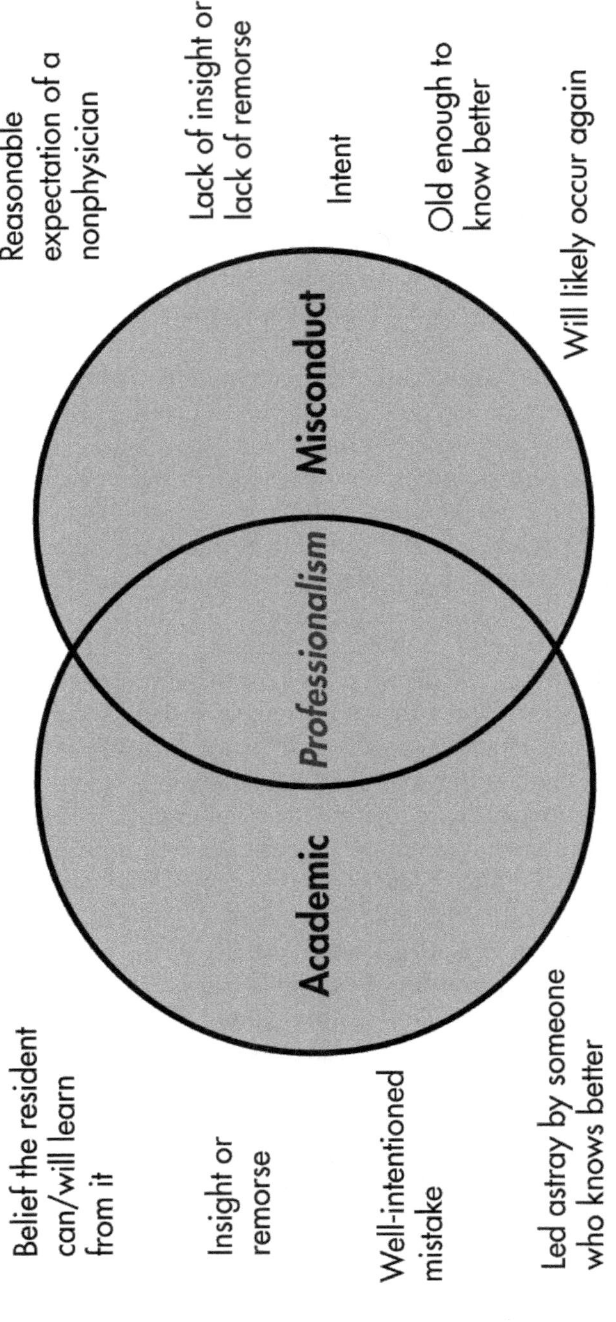

Figure 18.1 Venn diagram showing the overlap between professionalism and misconduct, with factors driving each.

Source. Frohna JG, Padmore JS: Assessment of professionalism in the graduate medical education environment. J Grad Med Educ 13(2 Suppl):81–85, 2021. Reproduced with permission.

a court trial; the process should gather as much information as possible to make the best possible conclusion and decision.

> When presented with the allegations made by the patient, Sam denied everything and said the patient was the one approaching him, but he rejected all invitations for communication or in-person contact outside of the care setting. In this situation, an inquiry will need to take place to determine the facts. An inquiry may include obtaining more information from the patient or Sam (e.g., texts or emails), speaking with others who may have firsthand knowledge of what has occurred, or following up with any other information provided by either party to the situation. If instead, Sam had not denied any of the allegations, an inquiry may not have been necessary. If he admitted to the allegations against him, then the school would proceed with appropriate discipline, which may include dismissal for misconduct. Even if Sam showed insight and learning from the situation, allowing him to stay enrolled and potentially engage in the same or similar behavior with another patient may not be a risk that the school or the health care facility is willing to take.

Application of Laws Specific to Student Health

Medical school can be stressful for students, and they may not always have the ability to identify and manage their own personal health issues. Student mental health concerns can manifest in several forms including depression, anxiety, and mental stress, especially compared with their peers. Recent data show that the prevalence of common mental health disorders among medical students are 7%–88% for anxiety, 7%–86% for burnout, 11%–66.5% for depression, 29.6%–49.9% for stress, 3%–53.9% for suicidal ideation, and 3.8% for obsessive-compulsive disorder (Aljuwaiser et al. 2024). Another estimation for suicidal ideation rates among medical students is 11% (Rotenstein et al. 2016). Medical school leaders are very aware of these increasing rates, which can cause ethical dilemmas for medical school leaders and faculty, especially physicians, who want to care for students and balance their concerns with the parameters of the law.

The Americans With Disabilities Act of 1990 (ADA) (42 U.S.C. § 12101 et seq.) is intended to allow individuals to decide what they want to share about their personal health information with others, including schools and employers. Simply stated, the ADA means that each person has the right to keep their personal medical information private. Regardless of health, however, all students should be held accountable to the same academic performance standards. Students have two choices: Keep the medical issue private and refuse accommodation/discrimination protections, or disclose and seek accommodation and protection from discrimination. Schools, like employers, may not solicit information concerning disability, which includes mental health diagnoses (Reichgott 1998). Despite its formalization in 1992, at least one study from 2016 concluded that most medical schools do not support the provision of reasonable accommodations for students with disabilities as intended by the ADA (Zazove et al. 2016).

When a student discloses a medical issue to a faculty member, that faculty member (an agent of the school) has an obligation to disclose this information to the appropriate school official. When a health issue is disclosed by the student, the school has an obligation to review and provide appropriate accommodations. The school cannot require a student to accept an accommodation but can choose which accommodations to provide if more than one would be effective; however, a university need not make any accommodation that would cause the institution "undue burden" (Association of American Medical Colleges 1993), meaning significant difficulty or expense. This is a subjective standard and varies depending on the resources, structure, and size of the institution. For example, a hearing impaired student may ask for an interpreter to accompany them to lectures or in the clinical setting. However, the school may determine that a computer-assisted device may be an effective accommodation instead, at a lower cost to the institution. It is ultimately the decision of the school, based on an interactive dialogue with the student, to determine an effective accommodation.

Conflation of a medical school's roles as both educators and providers of health care is often the underlying source of complexity and confusion around issues of privacy, communication, and evaluation of performance. Additionally, there is confusion among many clinical leaders serving in medical school administrative roles regarding academic law and employment law and how laws are applied to medical students, residents and fellows, and faculty.

Following several sessions with the Student Health therapist, Abigail (introduced earlier) continues to struggle and fails several basic science examinations. Worried about failure of first year, they meet with the dean and disclose their diagnosis and therapy. They request to retake the failed examinations with additional time allowed. Accommodations cannot be retroactively imposed in an effort to correct deficient performance; accommodation requests are to accommodate future performance, allowing the individual the ability to achieve the same standard as a student without a covered disability. Abigail's accommodation request for more time to take future tests must be evaluated by the university to determine whether this is a covered accommodation that is reasonable to help them to be successful.

Because Abigail was treated in a University-operated health center, and continues to be enrolled as a student at that University, HIPAA does not apply to their records. Instead, FERPA covers Abigail's personal health information and records and does allow for the Student Health Center to share their clinical information with others who have a need to know, even without Abigail's consent. Despite this allowance by FERPA, most schools have written policies that restrict this allowable practice. Students, faculty, and administrators should be familiar with their school's policies and practices. Additional common health scenarios are outlined in Table 18.2.

Discussion and Conclusions

The complexities of the law can pose various ethical and operational challenges for medical students and medical school faculty and leaders. This chapter provides a basic overview of common laws and regulations impacting medical student education, but it is important for medical school faculty to understand their respective school's policies and state and local laws. Navigating actions specific to student performance or health must incorporate applicable laws as well as a school's specific policies and procedures.

Faculty are encouraged to seek direction from the Dean's office or other appropriate leaders who are experienced with managing these issues on a regular basis.

Key Points

- Ethicolegal issues involving the oversight and management of medical students fall into two main categories: student performance (which includes academic performance and behavior/conduct) and student health.

Table 18.2 Common student health scenarios involving faculty

Scenario	Approach
Following a psychiatry lecture on depression, a student approaches the faculty lecturer to say they identified strongly with the lecture and believe they have depression. The student asks for a referral for evaluation and treatment. Should the faculty member provide this information to one of the school's deans or administrative leaders?	It is acceptable for the faculty member to provide referral options to the student. It is always best if the student can see a treating provider who is not a faculty member. If that is not possible or the student requests a faculty member, it should be someone who will not be involved with teaching or evaluation of the student. The faculty member should not share this information with anyone, including the school's leadership.
Following the lecture, a student asks the faculty member for advice on treatment of their depression: if they should try psychotherapy first, or perhaps start with a prescription for an antidepressant. How should the faculty member respond?	It would be inappropriate for the faculty member to provide any clinical advice to the student. They should focus on helping the student find an appropriate provider to make an appointment.
During a clinical rotation, a psychiatry faculty member observes a student who appears depressed and asks the student if they are OK. Is it acceptable for a physician faculty member to ask the student a few questions to see if, in fact, they may be depressed?	No. Faculty members (regardless of their expertise) should not engage with a student to diagnose or otherwise clinically evaluate. This crosses an ethical boundary between supervisor and physician.
A psychiatry faculty member has an established physician–patient relationship with an individual who is now a medical student at their respective school. Is there any reason the faculty member should disclose this to anyone?	It is inappropriate for a physician faculty member to both treat an individual who they will supervise or assess for academics. The faculty member should either refer the individual to another person who is not faculty for care or recuse themselves from supervision, feedback, and grading of the student.

- Specific federal laws and regulations (in addition to any state-specific regulations or institution-specific policies and procedures) must be followed when dealing with ethicolegal issues involving students.
- Educators facing potential ethicolegal issues related to a student's performance or health should seek direction from the dean's office or other leadership.

References

Aljuwaiser S, Brazzelli M, Arain I, Poobalan A: Common mental health problems in medical students and junior doctors—an overview of systematic reviews. J Ment Health 33(6):779–815, 2024 37933550

Association of American Medical Colleges: The Americans With Disabilities Act (ADA) and the Disabled Student in Medical School: Guidelines for Medical Schools. AAMC, 1993. Available at: http://files.eric.ed.gov/fulltext/ED370491.pdf. Accessed May 20, 2025.

Board of Curators of the University of Missouri v. Horowitz. 435 U.S. 78, 98 (S Ct 948 1978)

Board of Regents of the University of Michigan v. Ewing. 474 U.S. 214, 106 (S Ct 507 1985)

Daggett LM: The myth of student medical privacy. Harv L Pol'y Rev 14:467, 2019

Frohna JG, Padmore JS: Assessment of professionalism in the graduate medical education environment. J Grad Med Educ 13(2 Suppl):81–85, 2021 33936538

Minicucci RF, Lewis BF: Trouble in academia: ten years of litigation in medical education. Acad Med 78(10)(Suppl):S13–S15, 2003 14557083

Reichgott MJ: The disabled student as undifferentiated graduate: a medical school challenge. JAMA 279(1):79, 1998 9424050

Rotenstein LS, Ramos MA, Torre M, et al: Prevalence of depression, depressive symptoms, and suicidal ideation among medical students: a systematic review and meta-analysis. JAMA 316(21):2214–2236, 2016 27923088

U.S. Department of Education: What is FERPA? DOE, n.d. Available at: https://studentprivacy.ed.gov/faq/what-ferpa. Accessed July 16, 2024.

Zazove P, Case B, Moreland C, et al: U.S. medical schools' compliance with the Americans With Disabilities Act: findings from a national study. Acad Med 91(7):979–986, 2016 26796093

19

Diversity, Equity, and Inclusion in Psychiatric Education

Poh Choo How, M.D., Ph.D.
Ruth S. Shim, M.D., M.P.H.

Undergraduate psychiatric education (UPE) plays an instrumental role in the diversification of the psychiatric workforce to meet the mental health needs of diverse populations that have been historically excluded, marginalized, and underserved. Recruitment of students from backgrounds that are underrepresented in medicine (URM) is an important factor that contributes to the diversity of the future psychiatric workforce. Integration of cultural psychiatry, cultural humility, and health equity topics into formal preclinical and clinical curricula can support the interests of students in pursuing a career in psychiatry and develop the knowledge, skills, and attitudes needed to serve diverse populations. Leaders in UPE should be proactive in the recruitment, mentorship, and sponsorship of URM students with interests in psychiatry while also addressing issues such as mistreatment, biases, and inequities in grading, and other structural barriers that disproportionately affect URM students. It is important to address the (mis)treatment of psychiatric patients in clinical settings where the hidden curriculum affects students' perceptions of the clinical practice of psychiatry and where they are exposed to the impact of stigma, social determinants of health, trauma, structural (in)competency, and racism in medicine on the ability of health systems to provide adequate and equitable mental health care. Finally, partnership with leaders in graduate psychiatric education is imperative, given the roles that residents play in medical student education and the roles of program directors in the selection of psychiatric trainees. A shift from metrics-weighted evaluations to a holistic review process will further support diversity and inclusion in psychiatric education and training. The work of achieving diversity and inclusion in UPE belongs to all educators and should not be the burden of URM psychiatrists alone.

Recruitment and Retention of URM Students

Recent data from the Association of American Medical Colleges (AAMC) indicate ongoing disparities in acceptance rates of URM students into U.S. medical colleges. In 2022, acceptance rates for Asian, Latinx/Hispanic, and White applicants (46%, 47%, and 44% respectively) were comparable to the overall acceptance rate of 43% for all applicants, whereas African American and Black applicants were accepted at a lower rate of 39% (Association of American Medical Colleges 2022). Additionally, first-generation students who are the first in their families to attend college made up only 11% of those accepted into medical colleges. Data around graduation rates from American medical colleges show even greater inequities, with 49% and 24% of 2022 graduates (i.e., a total of three-quarters of graduates) identifying as White and Asian, respectively; only 7% of graduates identified as Black or African American, and only 6% were from Latinx and Hispanic backgrounds. (Data based on sexual orientation, gender identification, and disability status are not available, although it is important to consider how inequities along these lines—as well as the intersectionality of these various identities—affect the rates of acceptance, matriculation, and graduation.)

To address these inequities, greater attention and resources should be committed during premedical education to encourage students from URM and first-generation backgrounds (particularly first-generation, low-income [FGLI] students) to consider careers in medicine and to support their trajectory toward matriculation into medical colleges. URM and FGLI students face numerous barriers in pursuing careers in medicine such as strained personal resources and limited early exposure to clinical experiences, in part owing to a lack of networking opportunities and limited access to guidance and mentoring from URM physicians who are themselves underrepresented among practicing physicians (Freeman et al. 2016). Pathway programs can help students navigate the prehealth terrain and provide mentorship and opportunities for research and clinical experiences that increase their competitiveness in the medical school application process (Stewart et al. 2020). Some successful pathway programs begin as early as elementary school; others provide alternate pathways to medical schools including bachelor's-doctorate (BS-MD) programs, community college to medical school pathways, and postbaccalaureate programs (Parsons et al. 2022). Near-peer mentorship (such as pairing medical student mentors with high school students from lower income and URM backgrounds) can increase interest in pursuing a pre–health care career track (Patel et al. 2015). Leaders in UPE should consider being involved or involving psychiatric trainees in the mentorship and recruitment of prehealth students into medicine and psychiatry.

At the same time, AAMC has encouraged medical schools to shift their application review processes to holistic review. Historically, greater weight has been placed on metrics such as grade point average (GPA) and Medical College Admission Test (MCAT) scores, which favor White and other privileged applicants who have access to test-taking preparation courses and other resources; these multiple-choice-format standardized tests are also biased toward specific learning styles (Arbuthnot 2017). Many URM and FGLI applicants and applicants with disabilities are screened out by these criteria alone. Alternatively, holistic review considers applicants' experiences, attributes, and the disadvantages they have overcome to obtain a college degree (Witzburg and Sondheimer 2013). An applicant with low economic resources may have had to work to support their family and pay for their own education being enrolled full-time in college. Such an applicant may have a low or failing score on standardized tests but will have developed invaluable experiences and intangible attributes such as self-sufficiency, resourcefulness, resilience, and tenacity that make them highly successful medical students, trainees, and physicians. Faculty, students, and staff involved in admissions should undergo formal training in the process of holistic review and in understanding implicit biases to reduce discrimination against URM and FGLI students in the admissions process.

Attention should be given to the retention of URM students by providing educational, financial, and other support as well as protection from bias and discrimination that disproportionately affect them. Medical students from URM and low-income backgrounds and those who grew up in underresourced neighborhoods are more likely to experience attrition, defined as withdrawal or dismissal from medical school for any reason (Nguyen et al. 2022). Based on 2014–2016 data on matriculants of allopathic medical schools, 2.8% of overall medical students experienced attrition. Comparatively, Hispanic (5.2%), Black (5.7%), and Indigenous (11%) students were more likely to experience attrition compared with White students (2.3%). Students from low-income backgrounds (4.2%) were also more likely to experience attrition versus those without low-income status (2.3%). The rate of attrition from medical school increased with each intersection of a marginalized identity (URM, low income, or from an underresourced neighborhood). These differences could not be accounted for by a lack of preparedness for the academic rigor of medical school, because the authors standardized MCAT scores in their analyses. Similarly, according to 2016 and 2017 AAMC Graduation Questionnaire data, medical students from marginalized identities assessed by the questionnaire (female, racially or ethnically minoritized, lesbian, gay, or bisexual students) reported more mistreatment and discrimination and experienced more burnout during medical school (Teshome et al. 2022). We discuss strategies to address these disparities in the following sections.

Curriculum

Most students matriculating into medical schools have not had prior experience of psychiatry as a field of medicine. Students entering medical school are often exposed to stigma about becoming a psychiatrist, and those entering medical school with an interest in psychiatry may also be stigmatized because of their interest in the field (Lyons 2013). Additionally, health care professionals and students have stigmatized attitudes toward people with mental illness comparable to those of the general public (Masedo et al. 2021). Early intervention through preclinical curriculum design and implementation that supports the inclusion of diverse experiences and perspectives has the potential to decrease stigma against people with mental illness and influence attitudes of medical students toward psychiatry in general and as a career. In addition to knowledge about psychopathology and treatments of mental illnesses, students need to develop skills and attributes such as cultural humility to work with diverse and marginalized patient populations, including people with mental illness.

Cultural humility is a framework that adopts a lifelong commitment to self-reflection and critique while maintaining awareness of power imbalances in the physician–patient dynamic, with an emphasis on the importance of advocating for and engaging with communities (Tervalon and Murray-García 1998). Cultural humility calls for providers to approach clinical encounters with an attitude of curiosity and openness and a willingness to learn from the patient. It also emphasizes the awareness of the power differential between patient and provider, which has significant implications in the practice of psychiatry—for example, in the involuntary hospitalization of patients.

Topics such as cultural humility and cultural psychiatry have often been considered fringe or niche topics and not given adequate time and attention in UPE curricula. This attitude has the potential to exclude the experiences of URM, LGBTQ, and other underrepresented groups as they recognize the dissonance between what is emphasized in their curriculum versus their own experiences and the experiences of their communities. Alternatively, the willingness to highlight shameful diagnostic and clinical errors in psychiatry—such as drapetomania (a "psychological disorder" attributed to enslaved Black people who ran away from captivity), the pathologizing of homosexuality, the overdiagnosis of schizophrenia in African Americans, and the psychopathologizing of transgender individuals—not only models cultural humility but also can help students from URM, LGBTQ, and other marginalized backgrounds feel seen and included (Simonsen and Shim 2019). It is important to allow for deep exploration of topics such as social determinants of mental health, mental health equity, racism in mental health, and trauma and harms caused by the institution of psychiatry in the preclinical curriculum to prepare students to become advocates for future patients and communities they will serve. Students should also develop an understanding of how implicit biases contribute to racism in medicine and psychiatry as they prepare for their clinical clerkships.

For most medical students, the psychiatry clerkship will be their first exposure to the clinical practice of psychiatry and potentially the first time they care for patients with mental illnesses. The mental status examination (MSE) forms the basis of psychiatric evaluation and was formulated to be an objective measure of behavior. It is a very subjective tool, however, and is quite problematic when implemented without an understanding of implicit bias and the contextualization of patients' intersectional identities within the larger system. In research on bias, many typical observations made in the MSE have been commonly associated with specific minoritized groups, such as the attribution of lack of cooperativity to Black patients and lack of intelligence to obese patients (Chapman et al. 2013). In implicit association tests (IATs), both medical students and psychiatrists were more likely to pair Black individuals with psychotic disorders, noncompliance, and antipsychotic medications compared with mood disorders or antidepressant medications (Londono Tobon et al. 2021).

Although these attitudes may not be explicitly taught in the formal curriculum as facts, they are transmitted to learners via the hidden curriculum, where ideological and subliminal messages are communicated through human behaviors and the structures and practices of institutions (Wear and Skillicorn 2009). Elements of the hidden curriculum arise from the role modeling of attendings, residents, and clinical staff based on their experience and intuition. Learners witness how psychiatric patients are evaluated, treated, and spoken to and about, and they consciously or subconsciously internalize the same biases, beliefs, attitudes, manners, and patterns of interaction with patients. Students who suffer from mental illnesses such as depression and anxiety may be discouraged from seeking help if they witness patients with mental illness spoken of or treated disparagingly.

URM students who witness and observe the disparities in the treatment of patients from marginalized groups (e.g., Black, transgender, and unhoused patients) may develop a distaste for psychiatry as a field, which may negatively affect the recruitment of URM students into psychiatry. These experiences are not limited to the psychiatry clerkship alone. Discriminatory and inequitable treatment of patients with mental illnesses and substance use disorders by clinicians from all specialties contributes to the hidden curriculum and stigmatization of people with mental illness. Without the practice of cultural humility and awareness of their own implicit biases, attendings inadvertently contribute to structural racism and mental health inequities, as well as negatively influence trainees and students through the hidden curriculum. Leaders in UPE should formally and directly address the hidden curriculum through faculty development on cultural humility, implicit bias awareness, antiracism training, and structural competence, which involves developing competencies in the understanding and addressing of structural racism and mental health care inequities.

Addressing Grading and Other Inequities

Implicit bias and discrimination also play a role in clerkship grading inequities. Clerkship grades have traditionally been considered an objective measure of a student's clinical performance. However, these grades are determined by a combination of objective and subjective components including faculty and resident assessments and are therefore subject to the biases of the evaluators (Hauer and Lucey 2019). It is also difficult to standardize grading across different clinical sites and evaluators. A survey of fourth-year medical students at six institutions found that only 44% of students believed that grading was fair, and the majority of students believed that being liked by supervisors most influenced final grades (Bullock et al. 2019).

In February 2020, the cosponsors of the U.S. Medical Licensing Examination (USMLE) Step 1—the National Board of Medical Examiners (NBME) and the Federation of State Medical Boards (FSMB)—announced a transition for reporting a numerical score to a pass/fail score. This decision was based on recommendations from the Invitational Conference on USMLE Scoring (2019). The report cited concerns of equity and flaws in the transition from medical school to residency training as prompting these recommendations. These recommendations are consistent with existing knowledge that standardized examinations, like the NBME-style shelf examinations, have been used historically to exclude people of certain socioeconomic groups and racial and ethnic backgrounds from specific professional spaces.

Work is being done to quantify and address clerkship grading inequities in medical schools nationwide. In an internal examination of the association between race and ethnicity and clinical grading, University of Washington School of Medicine researchers found that White students were more likely to receive higher final clerkship grades compared with URM and non-URM students (Low et al. 2019). Further examination in this space has demonstrated, time and again, that inequities in clerkship grading disproportionately affect URM students. For example, women, URM, and LGBTQ students are more likely to report lower evaluations or grades based on their gender, race and ethnicity, or sexual orientation rather than performance (Nguyen et al. 2022). Small differences in the assessment of clinical performance escalate into large differences in grades and awards (Teherani et al. 2018). URM students were less likely to be given honors grades (less than 50% compared with non-URM students) or be selected for honor society membership (less than 30% compared with non-URM students). Racial disparities also exist in the selection of student membership in the Alpha Omega Alpha (AOA) honor society (Boatright et al. 2017), with Black (0.15 adjusted odds ratio) and Asian (0.52 adjusted odds ratio) medical students less likely to be members of AOA than their White counterparts.

In a move toward equity, some medical schools (e.g., Mount Sinai, Washington University, University of California San Francisco (UCSF), Yale, Stanford, University of California Davis) have moved from three-tiered clerkship grading measures (honors/pass/fail) to pass/fail grading for clinical clerkships. In place of clerkship grades, which feature performance-oriented learning models that emphasize ranking, time-based progress, fixed mindsets, and decontextualized learning, educators are promoting a shift to mastery-oriented learning models that promote learning by recognizing each student's capacity to learn, emphasizing frequent, immediate, and actionable feedback contextualized in the real world, learner-centered progress mapping, and adopting a growth mindset (Table 19.1) (Torre et al. 2020).

Based on the mastery-oriented learning model, in place of clerkship grades, UCSF implemented work-based formative assessments and feedback throughout the core clerkships (Bullock et al. 2022). Faculty were trained in providing real-time feedback and assessments, with

Table 19.1 Performance-oriented versus mastery-oriented learning models

Category	Performance-oriented model	Mastery-oriented model
Purpose	To classify and rank	To promote learning
Learner ability	Some will learn more and better	All have the capacity to learn
Feedback	Infrequent; correct/incorrect	Frequent, immediate, actionable
Progress	Time-based	Based on progress map
Context	Decontextualized	Real world
Mindset	Fixed	Growth

Source. Adapted from Torre et al. 2020.

emphasis on growth in the learning and clinical application of the subject matter over the course of the clerkship.

Mistreatment and Discrimination in the Learning Environment

Female, URM, and LGBTQ students are disproportionately affected by mistreatment including experiences of discrimination, public humiliation, and being the object of offensive remarks based on sex, race and ethnicity, and sexual orientation (Hill et al. 2020). Of students who reported being publicly humiliated during medical school, these behaviors were most attributed to clerkship faculty in a clinical setting, followed by a resident or intern. Most students who witnessed or received these behaviors did not report them; the top three reasons for not reporting were that they did not think it was important enough to report, they did not think anyone would do anything about it, or they feared reprisal (Association of American Medical Colleges 2023). Part of retaining URM, LGBTQ, and other marginalized groups in medical education is addressing mistreatment. This involves 1) developing a process by which students can report mistreatment and be protected from retaliation while doing so, and 2) implementing a restorative justice process as a way to repair harm from mistreatment of medical students (Acosta and Karp 2018). Restorative justice can help the learning community understand the personal and collective harms that have occurred and create conditions that incentivize those who have harmed or mistreated students to agree to be held accountable rather than deny or minimize the harm. At the institutional and structural level, health systems should adopt zero-tolerance policies against the mistreatment of learners and trainees in clinical settings.

Attention should be given to stigma and discrimination against students who have a mental illness and certain identities. This stigma and discrimination make it difficult for certain students to be successful in psychiatry. Many students report an interest in psychiatry due to experiencing a mental illness themselves or having a family member or close friend with mental illness or substance use disorder. Stigma and mistreatment due to mental illness can discourage their reaching out for care as well as any interest in pursuing psychiatry as a career. Often, medical schools lack support and accommodations for students with mental illness. In a survey of 1,428 students from 40 U.S. medical schools, one-third screened positive for anxiety and one-quarter screened positive for depression (Halperin et al. 2021). These rates were even higher during the COVID-19 pandemic. To ensure that all students, including those with mental illness and substance use disorders, are appropriately included in undergraduate medical education, schools should implement and enforce antidiscrimination policies. In addition, medical school administrations should work closely with institutional disability offices to make sure that students with mental health or substance use disorders have adequate support to ensure success in medical school, including accommodations for testing within the curriculum and for standardized tests.

Role Modeling, Mentorship, and Sponsorship

AAMC Graduation Questionnaire data suggest that the strongest influence on the selection of a specialty is fit with personality, interests, and skills (90%), followed by the content of the specialty (80%) and role model influence (50%) (Association of American Medical Colleges 2023). The most helpful resource, as cited by students, in learning about a specialty choice and career planning is advising and mentoring, followed by participation in in-house and extramural electives. Leaders in UPE should help to expose URM students to psychiatry as early as the first year of medical school, pair them with a mentor/role model, and increase opportunities to shadow and work with mentors in psychiatry, especially URM mentors. Leaders in UPE can help create opportunities for in-house and extramural electives and ensure equitable distribution of opportunities, such as travel stipends to attend a conference, engagement in research, scholarly opportunities such as poster presentations and publications, and sponsorship for awards and recognition. URM role models are needed, so leaders in UPE must prioritize the diversification of academic faculty in psychiatry. In addition to recruiting psychiatry faculty from diverse communities, we also must ensure that these faculty are supported and feel a sense of belonging when they are recruited. Retention and faculty development programs should target URM psychiatry faculty, and psychiatry departments should undergo well-facilitated training in implicit bias, structural racism, and antiracism to ensure that leaders in psychiatry are not creating toxic or harmful environments for faculty from diverse and historically marginalized and oppressed communities.

Residency Application and UME-GME transition

Support is needed to help students, particularly URM students, navigate the terrain of Electronic Residency Application Service (ERAS) applications for residency positions in psychiatry, which has become increasingly competitive over the last few years. Students need guidance on the number and type of programs to apply to, their personal statements, and selecting letter writers. Faculty also need to be trained in how to effectively write letters of recommendation. Residency selection committees should be aware of biases in clerkship grades, in awarding AOA, and in words used to describe female and URM students in letters (Khan et al. 2023), clerkship evaluations, and medical student performance evaluations (Ross et al. 2017). Historically, psychiatry residency programs have factored USMLE Step 1 scores into consideration of the quality of an application, with some programs even screening out and eliminating applicants from consideration because of a "low" Step 1 score. Now that USMLE Step 1 grading has switched to pass/fail, this is less likely to occur; however, unintended consequences of this policy change may lead to worsening discrimination against URM students. First, shortly after changing grading to pass/fail, the NBME also increased the minimum passing score, which had a secondary effect of increasing the number of students who fail Step 1, despite the pass/fail designation. As a result, residency programs might still choose to eliminate quality applicants from consideration if they have failed Step 1. Additionally, without a score on Step 1, which some programs mistakenly rely on to identify applicants, programs may move to assessing applicants using scoring on Step 2. Therefore, future consideration should be given to transition to pass/fail options for Step 2 (and Step 3) as well. Alternatively, perhaps a more impactful effort would be to eliminate the use of standardized examinations such as USMLE Step 1 and Step 2 as criteria for medical school graduation.

Conclusions

A multifaceted approach and longstanding commitment from medical education leaders are required to improve diversity, equity, and inclusion in undergraduate psychiatric education. Recruitment and retention of students from diverse backgrounds starts in the prehealth stage and requires the practice of holistic review, dedication of resources to support disadvantaged students, mentorship, and sponsorship from URM faculty from an early stage. Curriculum innovation is needed to develop inclusive curricula that reflect diverse perspectives and address the history of discrimination and racism in psychiatry through the integration of cultural humility, implicit bias, antiracism training, and structural competency in preclinical and clinical curricula. Actively taking steps to break down barriers for URM students in psychiatric education involves addressing the hidden curriculum, mistreatment, discrimination, and clerkship grading inequities. The rewards of these intentional efforts include a diverse workforce of psychiatrists and higher quality of care delivered to patients of minoritized backgrounds, ultimately directing the field toward mental health equity.

Key Points

- Recruitment of URM students into psychiatry should begin early, in the prehealth stage of education, through pathway programs that provide exposure to psychiatry and mentorship by URM psychiatrists to increase the number of URM students pursuing careers in psychiatry.
- The practice of holistic review increases equity in medical school and residency admissions by selecting candidates with distance traveled and experiences and attributes that help students succeed in medical training rather than relying on standardized testing that significantly disadvantages URM and FGLI students in the application process.
- Retention of URM students includes providing educational, financial, and other support, including protection from bias, discrimination, and mistreatment.
- Inclusive psychiatric curricula address stigma against people with mental illnesses, redress shameful diagnostic and clinical errors in psychiatry, and center the experiences of historically marginalized groups. This includes addressing the hidden curriculum, implicit bias in the mental status exam, and racism and other disparities in clinical psychiatric practice.
- Grading inequities during the clerkship disproportionately affect female, URM, and LGBTQ students and can be addressed by moving to a pass/fail grading system and a mastery-oriented learning model.

- Faculty development in cultural humility, implicit bias, antiracism, and structural competency principles is imperative to achieve diversity, equity, and inclusion in UPE.
- Recruitment and retention of diverse faculty in academic psychiatry is crucial in the diversification of the psychiatric workforce by providing more URM role models, mentors, and sponsors for students in healthcare pathways.

References

Acosta D, Karp DR: Restorative justice as the Rx for mistreatment in academic medicine: applications to consider for learners, faculty, and staff. Acad Med 93(3):354–356, 2018 29087964

Arbuthnot K: Global Perspective on Educational Testing: Examining Fairness, High-Stakes and Policy Reform, Volume 13. Leeds, UK, Emerald Group Publishing, 2017

Association of American Medical Colleges: 2022 Facts Applicants and Matriculants Data 2022. AAMC, 2022. Available at: https://www.aamc.org/data-reports/data/2022-facts. Accessed September 24, 2023.

Association of American Medical Colleges: Graduation Questionnaire 2023. Available at: https://www.aamc.org/data-reports/students-residents/report/graduation-questionnaire-gq. Accessed September 24, 2023.

Boatright D, Ross D, O'Connor P, et al: Racial disparities in medical student membership in the Alpha Omega Alpha Honor Society. JAMA Intern Med 177(5):659–665, 2017 28264091

Bullock JL, Lai CJ, Lockspeiser T, et al: In pursuit of honors: a multi-institutional study of students' perceptions of clerkship evaluation and grading. Acad Med 94 (11S):S48–S56, 2019 31365406

Bullock JL, Seligman L, Lai CJ, et al: Moving toward mastery: changes in student perceptions of clerkship assessment with pass/fail grading and enhanced feedback. Teach Learn Med 34(2):198–208, 2022 34014793

Chapman EN, Kaatz A, Carnes M: Physicians and implicit bias: how doctors may unwittingly perpetuate health care disparities. J Gen Intern Med 28(11):1504–1510, 2013 23576243

Freeman BK, Landry A, Trevino R, et al: Understanding the leaky pipeline: perceived barriers to pursuing a career in medicine or dentistry among underrepresented-in-medicine undergraduate students. Acad Med 91(7):987–993, 2016 26650673

Halperin SJ, Henderson MN, Prenner S, Grauer JN: Prevalence of anxiety and depression among medical students during the Covid-19 pandemic: a cross-sectional study. J Med Educ Curric Dev 8:2382120521991150, 2021 33644399

Hauer KE, Lucey CR: Core clerkship grading: the illusion of objectivity. Acad Med 94(4):469–472, 2019 30113359

Hill KA, Samuels EA, Gross CP, et al: Assessment of the prevalence of medical student mistreatment by sex, race/ethnicity, and sexual orientation. JAMA Intern Med 180(5):653–665, 2020 32091540

Invitational Conference on USMLE Scoring. Summary Report and Preliminary Recommendations from the Invitational Conference on USMLE Scoring. 2019. Available at: https://www.usmle.org/sites/default/files/2021–08/incus_summary_report.pdf. Accessed September 24, 2023.

Khan S, Kirubarajan A, Shamsheri T, et al: Gender bias in reference letters for residency and academic medicine: a systematic review. Postgrad Med J 99(1170):272–278, 2023 37222712

Londono Tobon A, Flores JM, Taylor JH, et al: Racial implicit associations in psychiatric diagnosis, treatment, and compliance expectations. Acad Psychiatry 45(1):23–33, 2021 33438155

Low D, Pollack SW, Liao ZC, et al: Racial/ethnic disparities in clinical grading in medical school. Teach Learn Med 31(5):487–496, 2019 31032666

Lyons Z: Attitudes of medical students toward psychiatry and psychiatry as a career: a systematic review. Acad Psychiatry 37(3):150–157, 2013 23632923

Masedo A, Grandón P, Saldivia S, et al: A multicentric study on stigma towards people with mental illness in health sciences students. BMC Med Educ 21(1):324, 2021 34092225

Nguyen M, Chaudhry SI, Desai MM, et al: Association of sociodemographic characteristics with US medical student attrition. JAMA Intern Med 182(9):917–924, 2022 35816334

Parsons M, Caldwell MT, Alvarez A, et al: Physician pipeline and pathway programs: an evidence-based guide to best practices for diversity, equity, and inclusion from the Council of Residency Directors in Emergency Medicine. West J Emerg Med 23(4):514–524, 2022 35980420

Patel SI, Rodríguez P, Gonzales RJ: The implementation of an innovative high school mentoring program designed to enhance diversity and provide a pathway for future careers in healthcare related fields. J Racial Ethn Health Disparities 2(3):395–402, 2015 26863468

Ross DA, Boatright D, Nunez-Smith M, et al: Differences in words used to describe racial and gender groups in medical student performance evaluations. PLoS One 12(8):e0181659, 2017 28792940

Simonsen KA, Shim RS: Embracing diversity and inclusion in psychiatry leadership. Psychiatr Clin North Am 42(3):463–471, 2019 31358125

Stewart KA, Brown SL, Wrensford G, Hurley MM: Creating a comprehensive approach to exposing underrepresented pre-health professions students to clinical medicine and health research. J Natl Med Assoc 112(1):36–43, 2020 31980210

Teherani A, Hauer KE, Fernandez A, et al: How small differences in assessed clinical performance amplify to large differences in grades and awards:

a cascade with serious consequences for students underrepresented in medicine. Acad Med 93(9):1286–1292, 2018 29923892

Tervalon M, Murray-García J: Cultural humility versus cultural competence: a critical distinction in defining physician training outcomes in multicultural education. J Health Care Poor Underserved 9(2):117–125, 1998 10073197

Teshome BG, Desai MM, Gross CP, et al: Marginalized identities, mistreatment, discrimination, and burnout among US medical students: cross sectional survey and retrospective cohort study. BMJ 376:e065984, 2022 35318190

Torre DM, Schuwirth LWT, Van der Vleuten CPM: Theoretical considerations on programmatic assessment. Med Teach 42(2):213–220, 2020 31622126

Wear D, Skillicorn J: Hidden in plain sight: the formal, informal, and hidden curricula of a psychiatry clerkship. Acad Med 84(4):451–458, 2009 19318777

Witzburg RA, Sondheimer HM: Holistic review—shaping the medical profession one applicant at a time. N Engl J Med 368(17):1565–1567, 2013 23574032

20

Career Development and Leadership as an Undergraduate Medical Educator in Psychiatry

Some Advice

Robert Boland, M.D.

Many medical residents, perhaps almost half graduating from residencies each year, aspire to careers in academic medicine. However, only about a third of those aspirants will have an academic career (Patel and Michelson 2017). There are many reasons, the most common being the income gap between academic and private practice careers (Straus et al. 2006).

This disparity between interest in academic careers and eventual career choice is most evident for clinician teachers. Most medical residents pursuing a Ph.D. or a research fellowship will pursue academic careers. The problem is in the rest of medical academia: those who might enter the field because they desire to teach or mentor trainees.

Academic medicine offers many benefits and the potential for excellent career satisfaction: it can offer variety and a chance for diverse experiences, intellectual stimulation, and the chance for generativity as one fosters the growth of the next generation of doctors (Straus et al. 2006). Although the challenges of succeeding in an academic career may seem daunting initially, it is possible to thrive and advance in your academic career, even outside research success.

In this chapter, I focus on academic development and leadership for academic faculty contemplating a career in undergraduate medical education (UME), thus a primarily nonresearch career. For those interested in research careers, there are many resources (Ionescu et al. 2017) and training opportunities (https://www.nimh.nih.gov/funding/training) available. However, there is less guidance for those pursuing a career in clinical education, and this path involves different skills, expectations, and leadership paths. What follows is a summary of observations and advice collected through the years while leading a seminar on academic leadership careers.

Understand Your Career Goals

Most of us have a unique approach to setting goals. Some approaches are very formal; others are less precise. One suggestion is to think of your goals in terms of what you wish your life to be in 10 to 20 years. It helps to consider the specifics of a career—how you want to spend your day—and not merely titles or achievements. In other words, focus on what you wish to *do* as much as what you want to *be*.

Base your career decisions on these goals. However, do not overly tie yourself to them; you will refine them with time and experience. It is best to reconsider your career goals every year.

For those wanting a career in UME, consider what excites you most about UME. Is it the chance to mentor medical students directly? To be creative and imagine new ways to teach and inspire? Alternatively, is it the chance to exercise your frustrated thespian skills for a captive audience? No reason is preferable to another. However, it will help if you inform your career choice with an understanding of your motivations, as different goals may lead to different careers. For example, those preferring direct teaching relationships will likely enjoy life as a clinician on a teaching unit better than as an administrator for an academic program, even if the latter position seems more prestigious.

Understand Your Institution's Promotion Tracks

Most medical schools have diversified their promotion tracks to recognize the different types of faculty. In past decades, most institutions had a single faculty promotion track that expected considerable research and scholarly productivity. This is less often the case today. Most institutions have some version of a clinician-educator track, and many subdivide that into primarily clinical and primarily teaching careers, all with their unique goals and expectations for success. Such a diversified approach is welcome, particularly because the trend in most institutions of higher learning is toward growing the nontenured faculty, sometimes called the *contingent workforce*, such that they now often make up the bulk of an institution's faculty (U.S. Government Accountability Office 2017). To leave such a growing workforce with no path to advancement seems a good recipe for institutional failure. The fact remains, however, that at many institutions, clinician-educators find it more difficult to be promoted than faculty in other promotion tracks (Keating et al. 2022).

In some cases, the problem is not the track but the lack of mentorship and guidance for faculty in a clinical educator role. Sometimes, a faculty member may not be motivated for promotion and is content to be, for example, an assistant professor throughout their career. However, promotion benefits faculty for several reasons, as most institutions tie faculty levels to salaries and leadership opportunities.

Thus, it is critical that faculty carefully read their promotion guidelines and understand the requirements for promotion in their track. Most medical schools offer workshops and career advice seminars to aid faculty in understanding these criteria. Equally important is finding a senior faculty member willing to mentor regarding promotion. Some institutions automatically assign a mentor; if this is the case, one should confirm that the mentor was promoted on the same track (or at least is familiar with it). If an institution does not assign mentors, the junior faculty member should seek a mentor from their supervisors. This mentorship is essential, because despite what a medical school puts into its faculty guidelines, there may be a hidden curriculum emphasizing certain types of clinical achievement that a new faculty member will best learn through trusted and experienced faculty (Lee et al. 2023). For example, a mentor may understand better than you how much your institution values teaching expertise as a necessary faculty skill.

Understand That Being an "Academic" Means Being Productive

For many clinical faculty, the bane of their existence is the insistence on scholarly productivity. In rough order of hierarchy, the types of productivity recognized by a university or medical school include grant-funded research, peer-reviewed papers, nationally invited presentations, and book chapters (Keating et al. 2022).

For faculty pursuing research careers, scholarly productivity is a natural part of the job, as we disseminate our research findings through peer-reviewed papers and presentations. For clinical teachers, the opportunities to publish or present seem fewer. Most journals prioritize data-driven articles, which requires some research and statistical expertise. Many journals no longer publish case studies, nor are they likely to publish opinion pieces, unless by an acknowledged expert in the field. Still, opportunities for publishing non-data-driven papers and other written materials exist (for instance, this chapter).

Many institutions also now recognize less traditional types of productivity. These include involvement on national committees, course leadership, curriculum development, and nontraditional media (such as blogs, podcasts, popular press articles, and popular books). Often, it is easier—particularly for junior faculty—to engage in these activities. Be warned, however: although many universities list such nontraditional productivity methods in their faculty promotion guides, the traditional types of productivity are usually valued more highly by promotion committees.

Although clinical productivity is not part of the traditional types of productivity helping toward promotion, most academic medical departments largely depend on clinical income (Saunders and Rice 2020). Given the essential role of clinical faculty, more academic departments are creating clinical promotion paths that recognize clinical excellence or leadership as a type of productivity. If being a master clinician is your primary goal, it may help to ensure you are in an institution that values your talents.

Decide Your Strategy for Getting Ahead in Your Career

As a member of an academic department, you are part of a team. Like any team, each member is unique and brings particular and necessary attributes to the team's performance. It would help to consider what you bring to the team. What unique attributes do you have as a UME expert? In thinking about this, you should be creative. For example, a good research team needs people with excellent research skills, technical skills, statistical expertise, or experience with grant writing. If they are doing clinical research, they need clinicians who can help formulate clinical questions and anticipate likely obstacles. If they are doing educational research, they need educational leaders who understand students.

Regardless of your unique traits, it helps to work well with others. This is a multifaceted trait that involves more than simply being likable. You should be flexible, generous, and occasionally be willing to extend yourself to a group even if there is no obvious immediate benefit to you.

Consider the Needs of Your Institution

Why did Sir Paul McCartney, a guitar player, play bass for the Beatles? Because he was one of three guitar players and they needed a bass player. As often happens in academic medicine, this short-term sacrifice was ultimately beneficial not just for the band, but for McCartney's career.

Similarly, an academic department has a finite number of educational leaders: usually, the vice chair for education, the residency program director, various fellowship directors, the UME director, and the clerkship director. Many departments combine the UME and clerkship director positions. There may be associate directors as well. You may wish to be the UME director, but you may first have to settle for another position, such as a course leader. All positions are essential, although departments may not value them the same. Regardless, doing an excellent job will identify you to the departmental leadership as a promising educator and make you more eligible for your dream role.

Collaboration Is Key

It is difficult to negotiate an academic career alone. More importantly, it is not desirable. One should see working with colleagues as a critical part of one's job. Locally, finding complementary talents for team diversity can be most beneficial. Nationally, it is best to find like-minded souls who can be your advisors and support group. Neither should be difficult to find, particularly as your colleagues are also looking for team members and peers.

Colleagues can be found in many ways. Some can be project based, such as when a particular project dictates the roles and talents needed. Other opportunities include collaborating around shared goals or visions (Lieff et al. 2020).

There are some keys to help you be the person others ask to join projects. Maintaining a practice of personal generosity is essential. Never try to take all the credit for a project. It is vital to recognize the work of your colleagues, particularly if you want to work with them again. In return, your colleagues will remember your generosity and reciprocate it.

Collaboration is essential not only when it comes to projects—fostering connections has many benefits. Often, career opportunities come not from one's close friends but through acquaintances or friends of friends (what sociologists call *weak ties*) (Callier 2022). There are many ways to make such acquaintances, including through colleagues or meetings. Remember that every collaborative project, even if unsuccessful, is a chance to form relationships with your colleagues.

Learn How to Request Help From Friends

It can be challenging to ask for help, even from close friends. Few of us succeed without help, however, and asking for help is a part of professional growth. When asking for help, it is crucial to be specific, give a reason for the request, and include an "escape clause" so that the friend can gracefully decline without affecting the relationship (Glickman 2011). Once a friend commits to help, it is essential to get specifics, particularly a deadline for the favor, as it is human nature to put off things that might be uncomfortable.

Although it can be awkward to ask for favors, helping others can be a mutually beneficial activity. Most humans are, by nature, prosocial in that we feel good after helping others (Keltner et al. 2014) (some psychologists refer to this as *helper's high*). Thus, although we may be uncomfortable asking for a favor, we can feel reassured that, in a way, we are also helping our friend feel good about themself.

Learn How to Negotiate for What You Want

Generally, medical faculty members do not know how to negotiate, yet they often must advocate for their needs. They must negotiate their salary, promotions, and whether to take on new responsibilities. Fortunately, many materials, both in print and online, teach negotiation principles. A classic work is "Getting to Yes," developed by members of the Harvard Negotiation Project (Fisher et al. 1991). A fundamental principle in the book is that the best negotiation outcome is *win-win*, in which everyone feels satisfied with what they gain from the negotiations. When approaching a negotiation, you can ensure that outcome by doing advanced preparation to understand your supervisor's or employer's needs and develop your asks in the context of the organization's goals.

Stick to Your Values

Working in an organization entails a compromise between your needs and those of the organization. When the two do not align, you may occasionally "take one for the team" and help your organization by doing something you would prefer not to do.

That said, you must first determine what lines you will not cross. Decide your core values and never compromise them, regardless of the potential gains. You may agree to cover a service to help a team member even though it is outside your role. However, you should never do things that compromise your values, such as gossip about or backstab colleagues, even if doing so might bring you some gain (for example, if you are competing with them for a leadership role). In the long run, sticking to values will benefit you: your colleagues will know you as someone they can trust.

One should be thoughtful in deciding one's values and limit them to those that are most central to your identity. Too many and you will be seen as overly rigid, uncompromising, and a poor team member. However, if you have too few, you should wonder whether you are giving enough thought to your integrity and reputation.

Consider Moving

Many academic leaders have had successful careers at single institutions. The leadership turnover rate at most institutions is relatively reasonable. Thus, waiting until a desired UME position opens can be beneficial. There is significant variation, however, and some UME leaders are "lifers"—having found their perfect job, they have no intention of leaving. Many academic leaders have found it helpful, and sometimes necessary, to change institutions to advance in their careers. This decision may be particularly true for more advanced positions such as vice chairs or department chairs.

In a large city, cross-institutional moving can be simple. Otherwise, a move may mean a physical one. Discuss the possibility of a move with a trusted (and discreet) adviser. Before leaving, consider discussing your dilemma ("I want a leadership role in UME, and yet there are no opportunities here") with your supervisor or department chair. They may have opportunities to offer that would keep you there. That said, do not threaten to leave as a negotiating tactic, as it is disingenuous and could backfire.

There may be other reasons to move. Academic medicine, particularly academic leadership, is still overrepresented by white males, especially at the highest ranks (Chaudhary et al. 2020). Many institutions are trying to increase faculty diversity (Powell et al. 2021), but diversity, equity, and inclusion (DEI) efforts have come under fire for political and other reasons (Finn and Kamerlin 2023). Some underrepresented faculty members feel saddled with significant responsibilities (e.g., leading their DEI programs) yet receive little support (Jordan et al. 2021). One hopes that all institutions will continue to find ways to promote equity in their faculty; however, if you believe yours does not and you fear unequal treatment, you may prefer to move rather than wait for change.

Involve Your Family

Before making important decisions, always discuss them with your loved ones, especially your partner. Career decisions you make involve them as well. This imperative is most apparent with career moves involving location changes or travel, but we may not realize how other career decisions affect them. For example, moving to a leadership position usually involves more work, which means more time away from home or interruptions during personal hours.

To succeed as you progress up the academic ladder, you will need your loved one's support. Involving your support system in career decisions will help ensure that support. This involvement includes the willingness to decline an opportunity if it presents too high a personal cost. Remember, no one lies on their deathbed regretting that extra faculty award they did not get.

Get Involved Nationally

For the young faculty member, national meetings can seem intimidating, and it can be challenging to meet new people in these groups, much less become involved. It may help to know that most other people at the meeting, including well-established members, often feel the same. For example, while leading one networking seminar at a national meeting, I asked the audience how many considered themselves introverts. Nearly every hand went up. This being the case, you can rest assured that many of your colleagues at a meeting also feel intimidated and will likely welcome your effort to meet them and hear about their professional interests.

Becoming a national leader is more straightforward than it may seem. The primary requirement for national leadership is a willingness to work hard without pay. National groups need volunteers to exist; not every conference attendee is eager to be one of those volunteers. If you are, that makes you a valuable person to them. Many organizations attempt to identify and recruit potential leaders through fellowship programs. These are excellent opportunities that usually provide travel funds and mentorship. They often offer chances for involvement, including committee membership.

We have limited time, money, and energy, so choosing which organizations to attend requires some strategy. There are often many organizations relevant to one's occupation. Initially, the larger conferences can be challenging to navigate, and it may help to begin with smaller groups. In psychiatry, the Association of Directors of Medical Student Education in Psychiatry is probably the most appropriate group, although organizations such as the Association of Academic Psychiatry include many UME experts. Many subspecialty organizations also have committees and content devoted to UME.

Getting involved starts with committee work. Some smaller organizations have open committee structures (i.e., any interested person can join). Others appoint their members. When joining an organization, you should examine their committee and interest group lists and choose a few that excite you. If the committees are open, attend their meeting. If not, look over the member list. If there is someone you know, or at least is from your institution, they could help put your name forward for committee membership. Getting onto a committee is usually not arduous, particularly in smaller organizations that are eager to involve interested members.

Once a member, volunteer for projects, follow through, and promptly complete the assigned work. In doing this, you are developing your reputation in the organization. When picking new leaders for the committees, the organization will usually look to the committee members who have been both productive and reliable.

A final word of advice for getting involved in organizations: show up. This advice has new relevance in the era of hybrid meetings. Remote workers who stay home all the time are less likely to be promoted than those who come to work most of the week (Bloom et al. 2022), and this trend is likely just as true for volunteer organizations.

Consider Formal Academic Leadership Training

In the past, becoming a leader was essentially a self-taught enterprise (Bronson and Perlman 2021). These days, many academic institutions have developed leadership training programs. If there is none at your institution, you can consider some national leadership programs available through institutions (for example, the Harvard Macy Institute, https://harvardmacy.org/) and professional organizations (Jeste et al. 2021). Most provide excellent training as well as networking opportunities.

Give Back

As you progress on the academic ladder, the focus should move from your own achievements to collaborative efforts that help others follow in your footsteps. Once achieving academic success, you can use your influence and connections to help your students and junior faculty. This is not merely a duty but a natural part of the academic journey. Ultimately, it is a joy: the most successful leaders take their highest satisfaction from seeing the success of those they have mentored.

Conclusion: Enjoy the Journey

As Arthur Ashe said, "Success is a journey, not a destination. The doing is often more important than the outcome." Although it is essential to have goals, a career is not simply about reaching the goal. Each step of the way contains unique challenges and opportunities for career satisfaction. One's highest position on the academic ladder may not be one's favorite. In the best case, each step will be fulfilling and prepare the way for the next. Whether one achieves one's original goals or decides on new ones along the way, the hope is that the journey will be fulfilling. It certainly can be. For a leader in UME, the chance to have a meaningful role in the development of thousands of future doctors can be an excellent way to spend one's professional life.

Key Points

- Understand your career goals
- Understand your institution's promotion tracks
- Understand that being an "academic" means being productive
- Decide your strategy for getting ahead in your career
- Consider the needs of your institution
- Collaboration is key
- Learn how to request help from friends
- Learn how to negotiate for what you want
- Stick to your values
- Consider moving
- Involve your family
- Get involved nationally
- Consider formal academic leadership training
- Give back
- Enjoy the journey

References

Bloom N, Han R, Liang J: How Hybrid Working From Home Works Out. National Bureau of Economic Research, NBER Working Paper Series, 2022. Available at: https://www.nber.org/system/files/working_papers/w30292/w30292.pdf. Accessed May 20, 2025.

Bronson B, Perlman G: The management experiences, priorities, and challenges of medical directors in the subspecialty of consultation-liaison psychiatry: results of a needs assessment. J Acad Consult Liaison Psychiatry 62(3):309–317, 2021 33092820

Callier V: A Massive LinkedIn Study Reveals Who Actually Helps You Get That Job. Scientific American, 2022. Available at: https://www.scientificamerican.com/article/a-massive-linkedin-study-reveals-who-actually-helps-you-get-that-job/. Accessed January 23, 2024.

Chaudhary AMD, Naveed S, Siddiqi J, et al: US psychiatry faculty: academic rank, gender and racial profile. Acad Psychiatry 44(3):260–266, 2020 32185748

Finn MG, Kamerlin SCL: Representation matters: responding to the current campaign against DEI efforts. EMBO Rep 24(9):e57850, 2023 37526390

Fisher R, Ury W, Patton B: Getting to Yes: Negotiating Agreement Without Giving In, 2nd Edition. New York, Penguin Books, 1991

Glickman J: Asking for a Favor: The Three Keys. Harvard Business Review, 2011. Available at: https://hbr.org/2011/01/asking-for-a-favor-the. Accessed May 20, 2025.

Ionescu DF, McAdams CJ, O'Donovan A, Philip NS: Becoming an academic researcher in psychiatry: a view from the trenches. Acad Psychiatry 41(2):293–296, 2017 26983418

Jeste DV, Patel S, Lee EE, et al: American Psychiatric Association's Leadership Fellowship Program: short-term and longer-term outcomes. Acad Psychiatry 45(2):142–149, 2021 33078331

Jordan A, Shim RS, Rodriguez CI, et al: Psychiatry diversity leadership in academic medicine: guidelines for success. Am J Psychiatry 178(3):224–228, 2021 33641375

Keating MK, Pasarica M, Stephens MB, et al: Promotion preparation tips for academic family medicine educators. Fam Med 54(5):369–375, 2022 35544432

Keltner D, Kogan A, Piff PK, Saturn SR: The sociocultural appraisals, values, and emotions (SAVE) framework of prosociality: core processes from gene to meme. Annu Rev Psychol 65:425–460, 2014 24405363

Lee CA, Wilkinson TJ, Timmermans JA, et al: Revealing the impact of the hidden curriculum on faculty teaching: a qualitative study. Med Educ 57(8):761–769, 2023 36740234

Lieff SJ, Baker L, Poost-Foroosh L, et al: Exploring the networking of academic health science leaders: how and why do they do it? Acad Med 95(10):1570–1577, 2020 31996558

Patel A, Michelson K: Why we need more doctors opting for academic medicine. KevinMD.com, 2017. Available at: https://www.kevinmd.com/2017/04/need-doctors-opting-academic-medicine.html. Accessed January 11, 2024.

Powell C, Yemane L, Brooks M, et al: Outcomes from a novel graduate medical education leadership program in advancing diversity, equity, and inclusion. J Grad Med Educ 13(6):774–784, 2021 35070089

Saunders EFH, Rice A: Between Scylla and Charybdis: a primer for navigating a department of psychiatry in the increasingly complex waters of academic medicine. Acad Psychiatry 44(1):106–110, 2020 31732884

Straus SE, Straus C, Tzanetos K; International Campaign to Revitalise Academic Medicine: Career choice in academic medicine: systematic review. J Gen Intern Med 21(12):1222–1229, 2006 17105520

U.S. Government Accountability Office: Contingent Workforce: Size, Characteristics, Compensation, and Work Experiences of Adjunct and Other Non-Tenure-Track Faculty. GAO, 2017. Available at: https://www.gao.gov/products/gao-18-49. Accessed January 11, 2024.

Appendix

The Teaching of Psychiatry for Undergraduate Students in the United States and Canada

Accreditation and Licensure Examination Implications

Marsal Sanches, M.D., Ph.D.
Michael McClam, M.D.
Robert Boland, M.D.

Medical schools and their graduates must meet certain standards regarding their quality and competency. In this section, we briefly discuss the requirements for medical school accreditation and medical licensure examination in the United States and Canada, focusing on their intersection with teaching psychiatry at an undergraduate level.

Medical School Accreditation

As mentioned throughout this book, the Liaison Committee on Medical Education (LCME), the body responsible for programmatic accreditation of medical schools in the United States, does not establish specific requirements or learning objectives for undergraduate psychiatry content. Still, in the Standard 7 section (Curricular Content) of the LCME Data Collection Instrument for Full Accreditation Surveys (Liaison Committee on Medical Education 2022), content from behavioral sciences is listed explicitly as a curriculum requirement (Standard 7.1). The curriculum should also include content and experience on different organ systems across the lifespan, including their implications for health care (Standard 7.2), allowing students to develop critical judgment according to evidence and experience (Standard 7.4) (Liaison Committee on Medical Education 2022). Other requirements include instruction on the medical consequences of societal problems (Standard 7.5), structural/cultural competence and health inequalities (Standard 7.6), medical ethics and human values (Standard 7.7), and communication skills (Standard 7.8) (Liaison Committee on Medical Education 2022).

From a practical standpoint, despite not being specific to psychiatry, these requirements become the basis for designing the psychiatric curriculum, at both the preclerkship and clerkship phases. Although schools have latitude regarding the content and specific topics to be formally covered, preclerkship and clerkship contents must be integrated with the school's established learning objectives and competency domains.

In Canada, the Committee on Accreditation of Canadian Medical Schools (CACMS) is the official body responsible for the accreditation of all medical schools (Committee on Accreditation of Canadian Medical Schools 2025a). As of this writing, all medical schools in Canada are accredited by both the CACMS and the LCME. In July 2025, LCME accreditation in Canada ceased, and the CACMS is solely responsible for the accreditation of Canadian medical schools. That change will impact Canadian students' eligibility to complete the U.S. Medical Licensing Examination (USMLE) examinations and to attend medical residency in the United States, as they will have to pursue Educational Commission for Foreign Medical Graduates (ECFMG) Certification. CACMS Standards and Elements outlines curriculum content requirements, which remain similar to those established by the LCME (Committee on Accreditation of Canadian Medical Schools 2025b).

Psychiatry and Medical Licensing Examinations

The USMLE is a series of three standardized tests required to obtain medical licensure in the United States. It is administered by the National Board of Medical Examiners (NBME). The first two examinations,

USMLE Step 1 and USMLE Step 2 Clinical Knowledge (Step 2-CK), are completed by students attending LCME-accredited medical schools in the United States and Canada still during medical school (United States Medical Licensing Examination 2025a, 2025b). Step 3 is taken by those who hold a medical degree from an LCME-accredited medical school (therefore, having already passed Step 1 and Step 2-CK) or certification by ECFMG, in the case of international medical graduates (United States Medical Licensing Examination 2025c). The Step 1 examination focuses on basic science concepts that are of importance for the practice of medicine, and Step 2 assesses the ability to apply medical knowledge, skills, and understanding of clinical science to patient care under supervision (United States Medical Licensing Examination 2025a, 2025b). Step 3, as the final examination, covers clinical situations potentially faced by a general physician, assessing the examinee's readiness to practice medicine without supervision (United States Medical Licensing Examination 2025c).

All USMLE examinations are based on an integrated content outline, and test questions are classified into one of 18 major areas according to the question's focus (United States Medical Licensing Examination 2024). Some questions are primarily related to individual organ systems, and others cover concepts of importance across different organ systems. In addition to medical and scientific knowledge, the questions are designed to assess additional tasks and competencies, including patient care (diagnosis and management), communication, professionalism (including ethical and legal issues), systems-based practice (including patient safety), and practice-based learning.

It is important to note that psychiatry-related content can be integrated into all major areas and competencies (United States Medical Licensing Examination 2024) to ensure students are well prepared for the USMLE examinations. For example, the Human Development area covers concepts related to psychosocial development, lifestyle, and coping strategies/stress response across the lifespan. The Nervous System and Special Senses area includes topics on neurocognitive disorders, delirium, and sleep disorders. Social Sciences covers themes related to communication/interpersonal skills and cultural competence, involuntary admission, and psychosocial aspects related to end-of-life, death, and grief. The content of the Behavioral Health area comprises syndromes and diagnostic categories inherent to the field of psychiatry, including psychotic disorders, mood disorders, anxiety disorders, somatic symptoms and related disorders, factitious disorders, eating disorders and impulse-control disorders, disorders originating in infancy/childhood, personality disorders, psychosocial disorders/behaviors (sexual disorders and gender dysphoria), and substance use disorders (United States Medical Licensing Examination 2024).

The Medical Council of Canada Qualifying Examination (MCCQE) Part 1 is the official licensure examination taken by medical students (Medical Council of Canada 2025). Students complete the MCCQE Part 1 at the end of medical school, and approval in the test is a requirement for admission into Canadian residency programs. The MCCQE Part 1 content is based on two components. The first, the MCC Blueprint, consists of four dimensions of care (Health Promotion and Illness Prevention; and Acute, Chronic, and Psychosocial Aspects), which are assessed across four categories of physician activities: Assessment/Diagnosis, Management, Communication, and Professional Behaviors (Medical Council of Canada 2025). These dimensions and categories directly or indirectly intersect with psychiatry and behavioral science contents, with the Psychosocial Aspects dimension of care corresponding to 10%–20% of the examination. The second component, the MCC Objectives, reflects the areas of proficiency expected of a medical graduate about to start residency and is organized into physicians' roles. Most objectives (which correspond to clinical conditions, complaints, and situations) are related to the Medical Expert role and include several psychiatric disorders, syndromes, and symptoms (Committee on Accreditation of Canadian Medical Schools 2022).

Conclusions

Although accreditation bodies do not list specific psychiatry requirements in the medical school curriculum, several of the LCME and CACMS standards are directly or indirectly linked to psychiatry and the behavioral sciences, making psychiatry an integral and indispensable component of undergraduate medical education. Moreover, to successfully navigate licensure exams, students must master key psychiatric themes and topics—an essential consideration in curriculum design.

Key Points

- Psychiatry and the behavioral sciences represent critical components of the medical school curriculum despite the absence of explicit requirements on psychiatry-specific content.

- Psychiatry and related subjects constitute an integral component of licensure examinations in the United States and Canada, thereby carrying significant implications for the design of medical school curricula.

References

Committee on Accreditation of Canadian Medical Schools: Studying for the MCCQE Part I. CACMS, 2022. Available at: https://mcc.ca/wp-content/uploads/medical-expert-objectives-en.pdf. Accessed July 28, 2025.

Committee on Accreditation of Canadian Medical Schools: About CACMS. CACMS, 2025a. Available at: https://cacms-cafmc.ca/wp-content/uploads/2025/02/CACMS-Standards-and-Elements-AY-2026-2027_FINAL.pdf. Accessed July 28, 2025.

Committee on Accreditation of Canadian Medical Schools: CACMS Standards and Elements Standards for Accreditation of Medical Education Programs Leading to the M.D. Degree. Standards and Elements Effective July 1, 2026 For Site Visits Scheduled in the 2026-2027 Academic Year. CACMS, 2025b. Available at: https://cacms-cafmc.ca/wp-content/uploads/2025/02/CACMS-Standards-and-Elements-AY-2026-2027_FINAL.pdf. Accessed July 28, 2025.

Liaison Committee on Medical Education: Data Collection Instrument for Full Accreditation Surveys. LCME, 2022. Available at: https://lcme.org/publications/. Accessed July 28, 2025.

Medical Council of Canada: Medical Council of Canada Qualifying Examination (MCCQE) Part I. MCC, 2025. Available at: https://Mcc.ca/Examinations-Assessments/Mccqe-Part-i/. Accessed July 28, 2025.

United States Medical Licensing Examination: USMLE Content Outline. USMLE, 2024. Available at: https://www.usmle.org/sites/default/files/2022-01/USMLE_Content_Outline_0.pdf. Accessed July 28, 2025.

United States Medical Licensing Examination: Step 1. USMLE, 2025a. Available at: https://www.usmle.org/step-exams/step-1. Accessed July 28, 2025.

United States Medical Licensing Examination: Step 2 CK. USMLE, 2025b. Available at: https://www.usmle.org/step-exams/step-2-ck. Accessed July 28, 2025.

United States Medical Licensing Examination: Step 3. USMLE, 2025c. Available at: https://www.usmle.org/step-exams/step-3. Accessed July 28, 2025.

Index

Page numbers printed in **boldface type** *refer to tables and figures.*